Dear Liz
expect miracles!
Laura Pañi King

Dear Cancer,

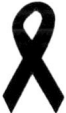

by
Laura Parisi King

Bloomington, IN 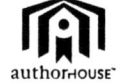 Milton Keynes, UK

authorHOUSE

AuthorHouse™
1663 Liberty Drive, Suite 200
Bloomington, IN 47403
www.authorhouse.com
Phone: 1-800-839-8640

AuthorHouse™ UK Ltd.
500 Avebury Boulevard
Central Milton Keynes, MK9 2BE
www.authorhouse.co.uk
Phone: 08001974150

All of the information in DEAR CANCER is based upon MY treatments, MY opinions, MY experiences, and MY understanding of medical procedures and terminology. It is not intended to be a substitute for professional medical help or advice. If you have or suspect you have a problem, you should consult with a healthcare professional. Laura Parisi King

First published by AuthorHouse 6/13/2006

ISBN: 1-4259-3244-4 (sc)

Library of Congress Control Number: 2006903496

Printed in the United States of America
Bloomington, Indiana

This book is printed on acid-free paper.

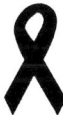

A Note From The Author

Two weeks after I was diagnosed with stage IV breast cancer I wrote a short note that said, "**Dear Cancer, you cannot defeat me**". Those six words gave me a feeling of strength and power at a time when I thought that all of my power had been taken away from me. I continued that note telling cancer WHY it could not defeat me, and before long I had turned those six words into a powerful message of hope and encouragement. I decided that if one message could make me feel so empowered, maybe I should write another and yet another.

I didn't plan on writing a book at that time. But after sharing some of my writings with people who were battling cancer and other illnesses, and seeing the emotions my words helped them to express, I knew that I needed to continue to write and to make those writings available to as many people as possible.

I found that it wasn't only people with cancer who related to my words, but also people with Lupus, MS, Diabetes and other life-changing events. People who were confined to wheelchairs and parents of children with disabilities also understood the fears, frustrations, outrage and anger that I wrote about.

In the course of writing DEAR CANCER I thought long and hard about whether I wanted to keep it a small book of inspirational writings, or expand it to include my story of being diagnosed with, and treated for, cancer. In talking with other men and women in various stages of cancer treatment I came to realize that there is no better way to support one another than by sharing our stories. Even though people experience this disease differently, there are feelings and thoughts that we have in common. Feelings of fear, anxiety and frustration. Thoughts of mortality and an uncertain future.

It is important to share our experiences with others as often as possible. We may never know how much our story might help someone else. Your experience with chemotherapy, radiation, finding an oncologist, or handling the after effects of surgery might be valuable to others. Your story might answer questions that someone else would not even have thought to ask. In turn, you might gain valuable insights from listening to others.

By sharing our stories openly and honestly, we give ourselves an outlet for our pain. We give ourselves the gift of being listened to and understood. We give ourselves the power to throw off our "victim" hats and become teachers, listeners, helpers and mentors. Most importantly, by sharing our stories we create unity and strength against an enemy that fights to tear us apart and weaken our resolve. It is my hope that DEAR CANCER will become a catalyst for unity and a source of strength.

It doesn't matter if you call this a self-help book, a book of poetry, or a memoir. What does matter is that you get something positive from reading it. Maybe it will help you to cry, bring you comfort, or serve as a validation of your own feelings. Maybe it will help you to feel less alone. Perhaps it will inspire you to write your own thoughts on paper. (I have provided you with blank pages at the end of part one if you wish to use them). It is my sincere hope that DEAR CANCER will give a voice to all of the unspoken feelings, and uncried tears. I hope that it brings you strength in times of doubt, smiles in times of fear, and hope in times of despair.

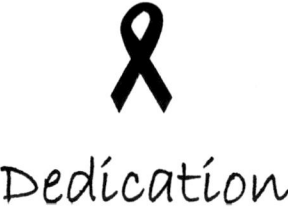

Dedication

Dear Cancer,

This book is for the hearts, minds, and spirits of those whose
Lives you have touched.

May their hearts find strength, encouragement, and support.

May their spirits find a gentle, yet firm, embrace.

May their minds find a quiet and calm place to rest.

May they know that they are never alone.

We all cry tears of anger, pain, and frustration.

We all have blessed moments of joy and happiness.

We all have "pity parties".

We all have suffered great loss.

We all fear for ourselves, and for our loved ones.

May those whose lives you have touched know that no
Emotion is to be judged as wrong.

May they accept their feelings with no shame or guilt.

May they cry rivers of tears, laugh until it hurts, and
Experience an abundance of joy, love, and happiness.

Part One

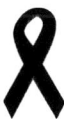

Dear Cancer

Dear Cancer,

You cannot defeat me !
I may cry, but tears are not defeat.
I may get depressed, but depression is not defeat.
I may get angry, but anger is not defeat.

You cannot defeat me
Because
I am more powerful than you.
I am loved…you are not.
I have friends…you have none.
People pray for me to live. People pray for you to die.
I have support, caring, compassion, friendship, and love.
You have none of these blessed gifts.

You cannot defeat me
Because
I do not fear you.
I feel for you.
For I will destroy you.
I will stamp you out of my life, and make sure that you are
Gone forever.

You, Cancer, will learn to fear me!!

Dear Cancer,

Some days I paint a smile on my face
Because I think it's what people want to see.

The old me,
The healthy me,
The "real" me.

The truth is…I'm losing touch with who the real me is.

My hair, which was such an important part of my looks, is gone.
I've gained weight because of the steroids that I have to take.
My fingernails are turning black and falling off.
My mind is foggy most of the time.
My quick wit isn't so quick anymore.
I don't laugh as easily as I used to.
My once athletic body is now filled with aches and pains.

I miss me.
The old me,
The healthy me,
The "real" me.

I know I'm in here somewhere,
But I'll be damned if I can find me.

Dear Cancer,

When I look in the mirror
I see the scars;
The constant reminder
That you have invaded my being.
I can't escape them.
They stare back at me
Each morning,
Each night.

                              When I look in the mirror
                                    I see my soul;
                               The constant reminder
              That I have the inner strength to survive.
                                You can't escape that.
                                    I will fight you
                                   Each morning,
                                     Each night.

My body may be disfigured,

But my soul is stronger than ever.

DEAR CANCER,

YOU ARE A PART OF ME.
I AM NOT A PART OF YOU.

YOU ARE JUST ONE SMALL PART OF A MUCH MORE
POWERFUL BEING.

YOU HAVE TRIED TO BREAK MY SPIRIT;
YET BECAUSE OF YOU I AM MORE SPIRITUAL THAN
EVER BEFORE.

YOU HAVE TRIED TO SHAKE MY FAITH;
YET MY FAITH IS STRONGER THAN EVER.

YOU HAVE TRIED TO INTERFERE WITH MY
RELATIONSHIPS;
YET THEY CONTINUE TO FLOURISH IN SPITE OF YOU.

YOU HAVE TRIED TO TURN MY LIFE UPSIDE DOWN;
Ok, you got me on that one.

Dear Cancer,

I control my sadness.

I decide if I will dwell on misfortune
Or
Plan a better tomorrow.

Complain about the storm
Or
Look forward to the rainbow.

Mourn the setting of the sun
Or
Enjoy the beauty of the setting.

If I control my sadness,

My sadness

Cannot

Control

Me!

Dear Cancer,

I cry
Because I am unsure of my future.

          I laugh
          Because I know that
          It is the best medicine.

    I pray
    Because I believe
    In the power of prayer.

          I meditate
          Because I know that
          Deep relaxation
          Is one of your worst
          Enemies.

I plan ahead
Because in my heart
I know that I will survive the battle,
And win the war.

          I smile
          Because I have learned so much
          About myself through my relationship with you.

          I survive
          Because I will not allow you
          To destroy my spirit
          Or diminish my soul.

Dear Cancer,

I used to think

That the more I gave to others,

The less I would have for myself.

Now I know that

The more I give...

The more I learn...

The more I grow.

Dear Cancer,

You have shown me that
I have so much
To be thankful for,
And
I have been wasting time
Looking at the negatives
In my life.

Dear Cancer,

You taught me how to smile,
How to touch,
Ignoring fear.

To laugh openly,
To cry freely,
To love,
And to
Allow myself to be loved.

You taught me how to find beauty, courage, and strength
Within myself.
To look forward to a new day,
To find peace in the night.

You will leave my body one day,
But you will be a part of me forever.

Dear Cancer,

I can make my future
Anything that I want it to be.

It is never too late
To start over,
To re-think my plan.

What do I want for my future?

What do I want for tomorrow?

Let's start with fresh fruit for breakfast
And take it from there.

Dear cancer,

Tonight I learned
What beauty there can be
In silence.

A friend and I watched
As the sun
Faded
Beyond the sand…

Beyond the water…

Beyond the horizon…

Lost in each other's thoughts,
With not a word
To disturb
The magic of the moment.

Dear Cancer,

People ask me if I believe in miracles.

I have seen the sun rise and set.

I have seen the night sky sprinkled with twinkling stars.

I have been awed by rainbows.

I have held a newborn baby in my arms.

I have sat on top of a mountain.

I have sailed over the horizon.

I have lived with nature in her home.

I have walked through forests.

I have pet manatees, and swam with dolphins.

I have watched a dog bring a litter of puppies into the world.

I have watched the ocean waves crash onto the shore.

Yes, yes I do believe in miracles!

Dear Cancer,

Since you came into my life I better appreciate each moment of each
Passing day.

You have helped me to experience the love of family and friends, (my
Love for them, and their love for me), in a way that I never had before.

You have helped me to focus on my dreams and goals, and on
Pushing myself to see them through.

Since you came into my life my marriage has been stronger than ever.
I have learned to appreciate myself, and the courage that I never knew
I had.

I love more openly. I cry more freely. I have more empathy for those
Who are in pain, handicapped, or suffering in any way physically or
Emotionally.

Since you came into my life I have learned how to pray. I have talked
To God, and remembered my deceased friends and family in my
Prayers. I pray _for_ them and I pray _to_ them.

Since you came into my life I have come to realize what a precious
And fragile gift life really is.

Since you came into my life I have started to live.

Dear Cancer,

I will not allow you
To have so much power over me
That I become bothered, or angered by your presence in my life.

I have complete control
Over how I choose to respond
To any given situation.

I have complete control
Over how I choose to respond
To you.

I will continue to dream
And set goals for myself.

I will continue to laugh at funny movies.

I will continue to plan events for next year,
The year after that,
And the years following.

I will look forward to my old age.

I will continue to have parties,
Go out to eat,
Go dancing,
Play games,
Be child-like and carefree.

Your power in my life, Dear Cancer, is limited.

My power
Is limitless!!

Dear Cancer,

Today I laughed out loud with friends and family.

Today I was inspired to write a poem.

Today I had lunch with my mother.

Today I went to see Christmas lights on people's homes.

Today I watched boats as they sailed around the waterway.

Today I kissed my husband and told him how much I love him.

Today I invited a friend over for the weekend.

Today I saw the most incredible sunset.

Today I enjoyed the warmth of the fireplace, and a good movie on TV.

Today I looked at old pictures, and got lost in fond memories.

Today I lived my life!

Dear Cancer,

You have stolen a part of me that I can never have back.
You have stolen innocence.
You have stolen trust.
You have stolen security.

Although a piece of me has died,
The woman still survives.

She breathes and lives
Despite your attempts
To suppress her growth.

Her beauty shines
More radiant than ever before.

She is the victor!
In spite of you,
The battle will be won!!

Dear Cancer,

I find comfort in nature.

The magnificence of the sunrise,

The delicate dance of trees swaying in the breeze,

The ripples that gently disturb the calm surface of a lake,

The welcome sight of birds in flight,

The relaxing calm at days end.

Nature heals my spirit.

It is my refuge,

My meditation,

My source of energy,
And
My serenity.

Nature is my home.

Dear Cancer,

No one needs to deal with you on their own.

Friends and family share our fear and pain.

Ready ears will listen if only asked.

Sometimes it helps just to talk it out.

No one will have magic words to make the hurt go away.

The magic is in the sharing.

Dear Cancer,

You are an invisible coward!
You sneak into people's lives unannounced and undetected.
You worm your way into the bodies, hearts, and souls
Of individuals and families.

You are a masked villain!
An intruder who sneaks into our homes in the darkness of night
Stealing all that is valuable and dear to us.

You are mysterious!
We never know who, when, or where you may strike.

Like all cowards you hide.
You hide within bones.
You hide within lungs.
You hide…afraid to show your face to the world.
Afraid to face the truth
That we are stronger than you.
We are stronger than you can ever dream of being.

You are weak and pathetic!

You are a playground bully!

You are friendless!

And like all faceless cowards,

You will be defeated!!

Dear Cancer,

I have started to get my affairs in order.
Please
Do not take this to mean that I have given up.
If anything
This process is making me even more aware of how important it is to
Fight.

As I look through my possessions to decide what I will leave to my
Siblings, my nieces, and my nephews, I think about each one of them,
And realize how very much I want to remain a part of their lives.

As I make decisions about the type of care that I wish to receive at the
End, I think about my husband. I think about all of the memories
That we have shared, and all of the memories that we have yet to
Create.

As I make arrangements for my funeral service, I think about my
Parents. I think about how they cared for me as a child.
I think about how unnatural, and heartbreaking it would be for them
To have to bury their daughter.

Cancer, this fight is not just about you and me.
There are many lives at stake here, not just my own.
On behalf of my friends, my family, and the thousands of lives that
You have touched over the years,
I promise to fight you
As long,
As hard,
As courageously,
As unrelentingly,
As fiercely,
(Do you get the picture yet?)
As powerfully,
As tirelessly,
And
As cheerfully
As I possibly can.

Dear Cancer,

I hate you!!
I hate you so much that some days I write your name on pieces of
Scrap paper,
Tear them up,
Stomp on them,
Burn them into ugly little ashes,
And flush them down the toilet.

Is that childish of me?
So what?
I don't care.

Because of you, I have resorted to uncontrollable crying and name
Calling.
I haven't done that since I was a child.

I wish that I could wring your stupid little neck, and stomp you into
The ground until you cry, "Uncle".

Man how I hate you!!
You're stupid,
Pathetic,
Cowardly,
Ugly, and mean.
You don't play by the rules.
You <u>have</u> no rules.
Nobody likes you.
If you were a real person your own Momma wouldn't like you.
That's how horrible you are.
You disgust me,
You pig-headed,
Worm-faced,
Puke-breath,
Crap-for-brains moron!!

Whew, I feel better now.

Dear Cancer,

You have given me an incredible gift.
You have given me the gift of insight;
Of viewing my life as it is in this present moment,
    Not 5 years from now.
    Not 10, 15 or 20 years from now.
But in this one single space in time.

I no longer view my life in years,
But in precious moments.

Moments spent listening to a waterfall,
Eating an ice cream cone,
Or reading quietly in bed at night.

Moments spent talking with my nieces and nephews,
Watching the sunset,
Or lost silently in prayer.

Moments spent listening to music,
Relaxing in a hot bath,
Or feeling the warmth of pajamas fresh from the dryer on a cold
Winter night.

Life is about moments.
It is about being present and focused on the here and now.

Because of you, Cancer,
I have come to realize that all I have,
All any of us has, is here and now.

Because of you,
I have learned to treasure every moment of my life,

            Without judgement,
            Without living in the past,
            Without worry about the future.

Dear Cancer,

The sun sets
And I am lucky enough
To experience
The sights
And
The sounds
Of the setting.

Dear Cancer,

I have no time for you right now!

I have vacations to plan,
Friends to visit,
And nieces and nephews to watch grow up.

I have books to write, and have published.

I have a marriage to continue to enjoy.

I have a boat to sail,
Games to play,
And nature to admire.

I have dreams that have yet to be fulfilled.

I'm sorry,
But I simply have no time for you right now!

Dear Cancer,

I will admit it
You frighten me.
I am afraid of the uncertainty of dealing with you.
I am afraid of not knowing how you will affect me tomorrow,
Next week,
Next year.

I am tired.
I am tired of the many tests and treatments that I must go through
Because of you.
I am tired of having bones that hurt night and day.
I am tired of the thought that you have entered my life.

I am afraid, and I am tired, but I promise you this;
I will fight you until the bitter end.
I will help as many people affected by you fight as well.
I will stalk you.
I will hunt you down wherever you live, and make your existence
Miserable.
I will starve you of everything that you need to live.
I will destroy you with my unrelenting faith.
I will hurt you with my visualizations and meditations.
I will abuse you with good nutrition.
I will diminish your power with laughter and positive thoughts of the
Future.

Cancer,
You have messed with the wrong woman!!

Dear Cancer,

I wrote the following poem to show you that my creativity, and sense of humor are still intact. No matter how hard you try, you will never take that away from me. You might take my hair. You might take my energy. You might even take my life. But, as long as I have a breath of life left in me, I will keep laughing, loving, and living.

THE ANSWER WAS CANCER

I once had two boobies, a pretty nice pair.
It took years to grow them, but I didn't care.
A matched set they were, rather perky and fine.
They sure weren't perfect, but they were all mine.

The mammos they gave me came back free and clear,
No lumps and no bumps, they showed nothing was there.
Then quite out of nowhere two doctors agree
That my poor little breast would need surgery.

Then a lump was removed, with a whole lot of breast.
The lump was then studied in test after test.
The answer was cancer, now I'll have to cope
With one breast a mountain, and one a ski slope.

"Stage II", they first said, so it's chemo, radiation.
My poor mind was swimming with pain and frustration.
"Now, wait! What is this? Your lungs are not clear.
It seems that the cancer cells have traveled here.

So now it's stage IV, "and, oh, by the way
Remember the bone scan you had yesterday?"
"We said it was clear, but oops, we were wrong!
It seems that the cancer was there all along."

"So forget about chemo, it's hormones for you.
We'll cut off your estrogen, that's what we'll do."

I now have hot flashes by day and by night.
Somehow at my age this doesn't seem right.

But alas, the old hormones did not do the trick.
The oncologist's words made me feel pretty sick.
He said I need chemo, and words that I dread,
"How fond are you of all that hair on your head?"

Out went the hair, every straight, golden lock.
In came pain, shingles, fatigue, chicken pox.
Eyelashes, eyebrows, and even the pubes,
Went to hair heaven to visit the boobs.

Wigs were too itchy, and scarves didn't suit me.
I'm tired and cranky, won't someone please shoot me.
Hot flashes, red rashes (I can't tell you where)
Suffice it to say, that the sun don't shine there.

Where this is leading, there's no way to know,
I'd like to tell cancer where it can go.
The bad times will come. And the bad times will pass.
Cancer, you can kiss my red-rashy ass.

Dear Cancer,

You have invaded my body.

I will not allow you to invade my mind
And my spirit.

I will not allow feelings such as hatred,
Fear,
Guilt, or shame
To take over my life.
I will not stoop to your level.
I view your presence in my life as an annoyance;
An inconvenience.
Don't get me wrong
I do have moments,
Even days when I get mad as hell.
But I will not become an angry and bitter person.

I have days when I am afraid,
But I will not become a fearful person.

I plan to continue on with my life.
I have always had a good sense of humor.
I plan to use it in coping with you.

I have always been upbeat and cheerful.
You can't take that from me.
My body is just the shell of who I am.
My mind, my spirit, and all that lies within,
Will continue to grow stronger each day
Secure in the knowledge that
You can,
And will,
Be defeated.

Dear Cancer,

I do not appreciate having you in my life.
I appreciate my life in spite of having you in it.

When I first heard that you had entered my life
I thought that my final days were at hand.
I thought that those days would be filled with tears,
Pain,
Anger,
Depression,
Loss of self,
Stress, and loneliness.

Instead, my days have been filled with phone calls,
Flowers,
Visits,
Cards,
Healing masses,
Words of encouragement,
Kindness,
Time for self,
Love of family and friends,
Generosity,
Spirituality,
Healthy eating,
Helping hands, and open hearts.

With each phone call that I receive from a friend
                    Your power is diminished.

With each night I spend laughing
                    You lose your strength.

With each healthy meal that I eat
                    You shrink and fade.

With each prayer that is said in my name
                    Your impact on my life is destroyed.

Dear Cancer,

I have often wondered,

How can something so terrible

Bring about so much good?

I think the better question might be,

<u>Why do we wait</u> for something so terrible

To bring about so much good?

Dear Cancer,

It is normal for us to feel fear when you enter our lives.

It is normal to feel anger,
Rage, hurt, and disappointment.

It is normal to cry.

It is normal to not want to get out of bed some days.

It is normal to look at other people and feel envious of their good
Health.

It is normal to be afraid to laugh for fear that it may be the last time
That you will.

It is normal to worry about the future.

It is normal to ask "why me?".

It is normal to not be strong all of the time, even though some people
Expect you to be.

It is normal to be sick and tired of needles,
Doctor appointments, and not feeling well.

It is all normal.
It is all OK.
People need to know that.

It is normal, and it's OK.
It really is.

Dear Cancer,

My life is, and will continue to be, different because of you.

That's O.K.

Who amongst us has not experienced pain?

Who amongst us does not have a challenge to face?

Who amongst us goes through life with no scars?

You, Cancer are my pain,
                  My challenge,
                                  And my scar.

As you shrink with each passing day,

I grow.

As you lose each battle against me,

I win the war against you.

As you become weaker,

I become a healthier,
                      Stronger,
                            More confident woman.

The more you die.

The more I live.

Dear Cancer,

Sometimes it's hard to think of myself as a breast cancer
"Survivor" while I am still entrenched in the heat of the battle.

Yes, this is a battle.
You have declared war.
I have gathered my ammunition as you have yours.
Let me tell you what you are up against.

I visualize ninja angels in my body.
These are masked angels who seek you out wherever you hide,
And bombard your pathetic, little cells with an onslaught of
Kicks and punches until they beg for mercy.
Keep begging.
The battle will rage until you are in full retreat.

I visualize housecleaning angels, who with their powerful
Vacuums suck your cells out of every little crevice where you
Hide, cower, and whimper.
They vacuum your cells from my bones, and from my lungs,
And throw you in the garbage where all the useless trash
Belongs.

I have construction angels who rebuild bones, and rebuild my
Body to it's healthiest state of being.

I have healing angels, who soothe my mind and spirit, and
Keep me feeling positive and optimistic.

I have the power of prayer, which is more powerful than any
Artillery ever invented.

I have friendship and laughter on my team.
I have meditation.
I have nutrition.
I have love.
I have hope.
I have dreams.

You have declared war.

The battle will rage until you are in full retreat, and I will be a Survivor after all!!

Dear Cancer,

I just came from the grocery store.
I walked up and down the aisles with my wagon.
I passed dozens of people, and not one of them saw you.
No one could tell that I am carrying you inside of me.

In turn, I could not tell what their inner demons are.
How many people looking at the melons in the produce
Section are suffering with life – threatening illnesses?
How many people in the checkout aisle are dealing with the
Loss of a loved one?
How many people in the parking lot are caregivers for
Parents, or sick children?

It made me realize that we need to be more gentle with one
Another because we have no way of knowing what the other
Person is dealing with.

Because of you, I now say "Does it really matter?" Over and
Over again.

"Does it really matter if I miss the traffic light and have to
Wait for the next green light?"

"Does it really matter if someone takes the parking space that
I was hoping to get?"

"Does it really matter if I burn a piece of toast and have to
Start over again?"

It really doesn't matter.
Wouldn't it be nice if we all came to that realization?
Wouldn't it be nice if we all came to realize that we have
Limited time on this planet, and that we are all struggling in
Our own way?

Wouldn't it be nice if we realized that by cooperating instead
Of competing the world would become a better place?
Wouldn't it be nice if we realized that it's the small gestures
That make the big difference?

Dear Cancer,

Some days I look at myself in the mirror
And it hits me,

I have cancer!
I really have cancer!!
What a frightening sentence.

It has taken me a long time just to say your name.
I have called you "the big 'C'",
"My condition", or "my illness".
It's as if saying the word "cancer" out loud would make it any
More real.

At some point I realized that you ARE just a word.
You ARE just a condition.
You ARE just an illness.

"I have cancer." IS a frightening sentence.

But it IS NOT a death sentence.

Dear Cancer,

I
Am
The
Most
Powerful
Force in my life!

Dear Cancer,

Because of you
I have seen
How much kindness
There is in the world!

Dear Cancer,

You are the unseen threat in a T.V. Horror movie.

You are the bullet from a cowardly assassin's gun.

You are the senseless ramblings of a madman.

You are a rogue storm at sea.

You are a blinding flash of lightening.

You are the essence of evil.

You are the silence that invades the night.

You are nothing and yet you are everything.

Dear Cancer,

I desperately search
For an unknown feeling,
A vague notion
Of what contentment
Is all about.

Now I know
It is about me.

I must make it happen.

Dear Cancer,

I will not allow you to darken my spirit.

I will not allow you to destroy my family and my marriage.

I will not allow you to frighten and upset my friends.

I will not allow you to rob me of my enthusiasm for life.

I will fight you with everything that I have.

I will use your strength against you.

The harder you push, the harder I'll push back.

You cannot win!!

Dear Cancer,

This moment,
In spite of you,
I feel
There is nothing
That I cannot achieve.

I am in control of my world.
All of my experiences,
All of my emotions,
All of my thoughts,
Are within my command.

I am the master of my world,
And
I master my world
With great pride.

Dear Cancer,

I am body.   I am mind.   I am spirit.

My body is a shell that contains the various systems that keep it alive.
I think of my body as a warehouse;
A place to store food, water, and blood.
I work hard to keep my body looking good because that is what most
People see when they look at me.
Am I fat?
Am I skinny ?
Do I have pimples?
It doesn't matter.
My body is not me.
My body is not who I am.

My mind contains knowledge,
Memories,
Thoughts, and logic.
My mind helps me to think and reason.
Am I smart?
Am I a fast learner?
Do I need extra help understanding math, history, or geography?
It doesn't matter.
My mind is not me.
My mind is not who I am.

My spirit extends beyond my body, and my mind.
My spirit is the essence of who I am.
It is my spirit that gives love.
It is my spirit that hurts when love is not returned.
It is my spirit that has compassion and empathy for others.
It is my spirit that soars when there is happiness in the world.
It is my spirit that cries at injustice.
It is my spirit that is in charge of all that's truly important in this
World.
It is my spirit that will lead the fight.
It is my spirit that will lead my body, and my mind, to victory.
It is my spirit that will not be broken.

Dear Cancer,

I believe that there are no coincidences in life.
I believe that everything happens for a reason.
I believe that we are spiritual beings who have been placed on this
Earth to have human experiences to learn and grow from.
I believe that significant others have been brought into our lives so
That we can learn and grow from their human experiences, while
They learn and grow from ours.
I believe that we must not wait until the time of our death to reflect
Upon what this life is teaching us.

<u>Now</u> is the time to look at significant moments in our lives, and look
For the lessons that we are here to learn.

Dear Cancer, what am I supposed to learn from my experience with
You?
What are others supposed to be learning through me?

I am learning to value every moment of every day.
I am learning to appreciate myself, and the talents that God has given
Me.
I am learning to neither live in the past, nor worry about the future.
I am learning to treat people with patience and acceptance.
I am learning to have courage in times of crisis.
I am learning that small acts of kindness go a long way.
I am learning that I am loved.
I am learning to love.
I am learning to ask for help when I need it. (We are all here to
Help one another.)
I am learning how important it is to share all of these lessons with
Others.
I am learning to look at others to see what lessons I am to learn from
Them.

I am learning that we are all in this life together.
We all have meaning.
We all have a purpose.
We all make a difference.

Dear Cancer,

You are my cross to bear.
You are my burden,
My challenge,
My test, and my passion.

I accept you into my life
Because it is through you that I am learning what true faith is.
It is through you that I am learning what courage means.
It is through you that I am learning to pray.
It is through you that I have learned more about myself than I ever
Imagined I could.

I now know that I can face incredible pain and suffering, and
Come out stronger for it.

I now know that I can maintain a positive attitude in times of
Despair.

I now know the meaning of friendship,
Loyalty, and commitment.

Dear Cancer, I pray for the day when the morning headline will read:

CURE FOR CANCER FOUND!!

Until then, I will continue to use you to **my** benefit.

I will use my experience with you as a way to put worry,
Fear, and frustration aside, and learn how to live my life to the fullest.

Dear Cancer,

This precious moment is all that I've got.

It's all that I'm promised.

It's all that I can be sure of.

It's all that I can count on.

It's all that there is.

Oh, how shall I use this precious moment?

Dear Cancer,

Does my laughter annoy you?
I can almost sense your frustration as I go on singing,
Dancing, and enjoying my life in spite of your existence.

Do you get upset when I ignore you?
I see you.
I hear you.
I feel you jumping up and down trying to get my attention.
Forget it.
I refuse to allow you to be the first thing that I think about in the
Morning and the last thing I think about at night.

Do I piss you off when people call to ask how I'm feeling and I say
"Fine"

"Real good"

"I'm doing great"?

Well if you don't like it,
Leave.
Go ahead,
Run and hide.
Go whimper off with your tail between your legs,
You big sissy!!

Dear Cancer,

Believe it or not, I don't blame you for what is happening to me. I'm
Angry with you, but I don't blame you.

It boggles my mind to think of how many chemicals we ingest, and
Put on our skin in any given day.

There are chemicals in shampoo, soap, deodorant, hair spray,
Cosmetics, lotion, perfume, detergent, and cleaning products.

There are pesticides, preservatives, and additives in our food.

There is carbon monoxide in the air.

There are traces of bacteria on shopping cart handles, restaurant
Menus, and doorknobs.

Who knows what is in the water we drink?
Who knows how I ended up with cancer?
Who knows for sure how anyone gets cancer?

No, I don't blame you. I'm not sure who, or what, to blame.
I don't even know if I can blame any one thing.

There is only one thing that I'm sure of. I have cancer.
I don't want to use my precious energy on feelings like anger, and
Resentment, so I will choose to focus on the things that I can control.
I will put my energy into learning how to relax, eat healthy foods,
Exercise, and take life one day at a time.

Dear Cancer,

I have chosen to take a new look at the chemotherapy drugs that drip
Into my veins week after week.
I will see them as life-saving liquids.
I will welcome them into my body as a healing force.
Yes, they will do damage to my healthy cells.
I will lose my hair.
I will feel tired.
I will not feel well some days.

But neither will you.
You too will get tired and run down.
You too will feel pain and suffering.
You too will feel loss.

This is my affirmation to chemotherapy. It brings me strength, and
Encourages me to keep up the fight.
May others who use it feel motivated to fight long and hard until the
Battle is won.

C hemicals
H elping to
E mpower
M e
O nward
T owards
H ealth
E nergy
R evitilization
A nd the
P ower of
Y outh.

Dear Reader,

The following pages have been left blank on purpose.

They are for you to use in any way that you want.

Feel free to draw, scribble, or write your own thoughts to cancer, or Any other challenge that you are facing.

Feel free to curse, cry, joke around, or be as serious as you'd like.

These pages are for you.

EXPECT MIRACLES

LAURA

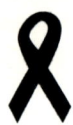

Laura Parisi King

Laura Parisi King

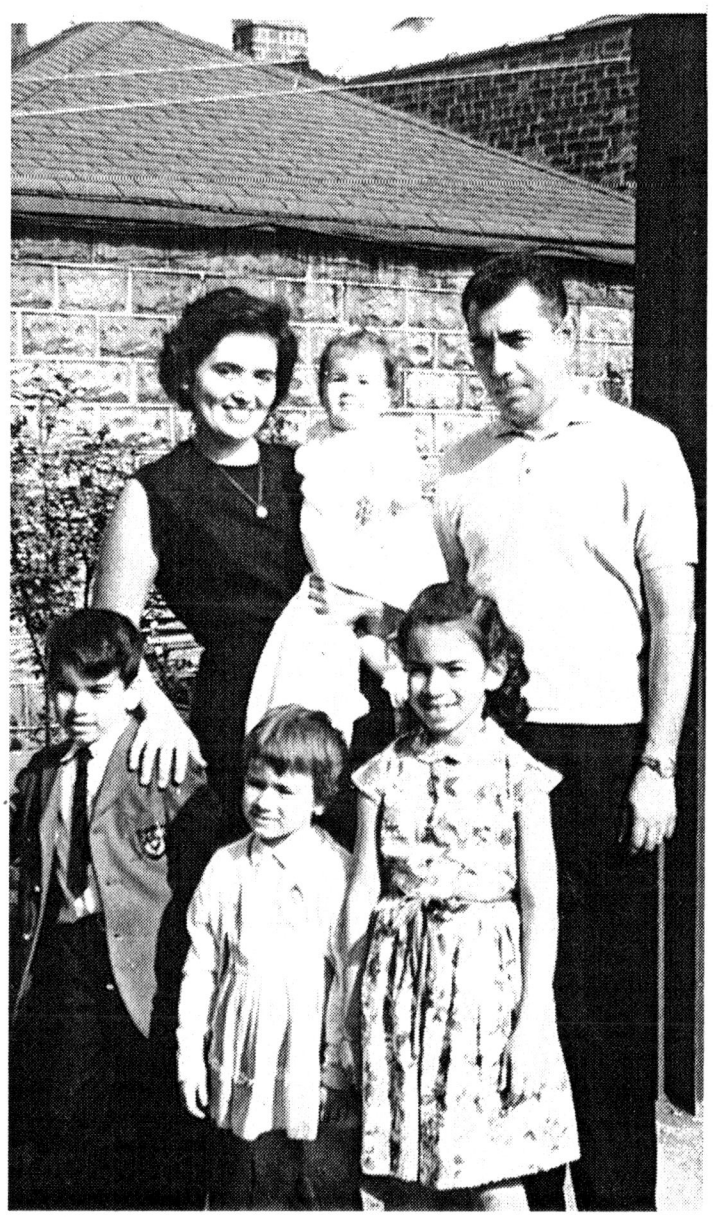

My mother (holding Grace), my father, George, me and Loretta, in
our backyard in Flatbush, Brooklyn. 1965.

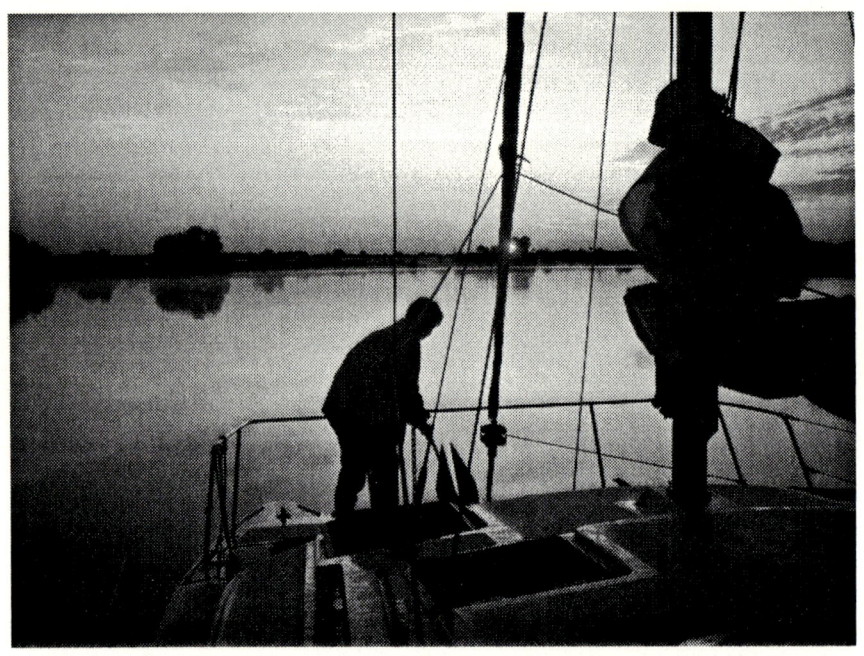

Peaceful mornings on the Intracoastal Waterway.

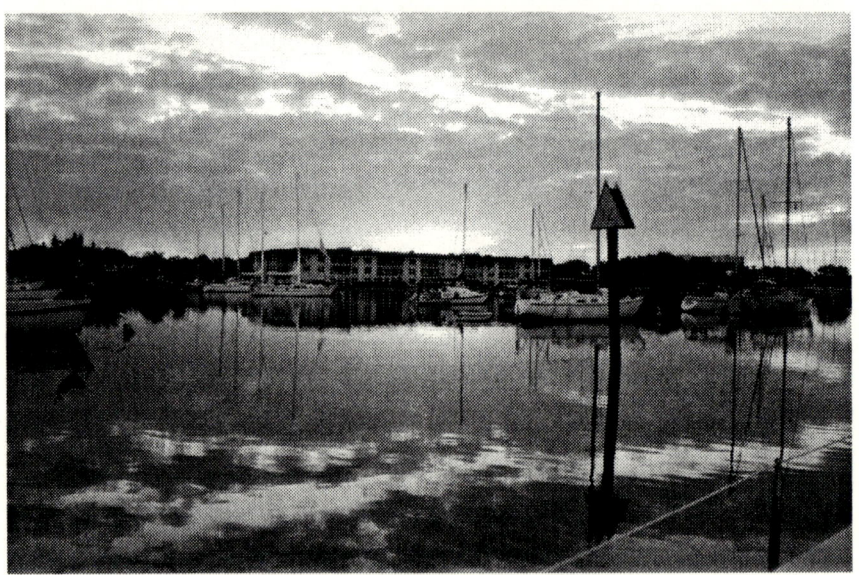

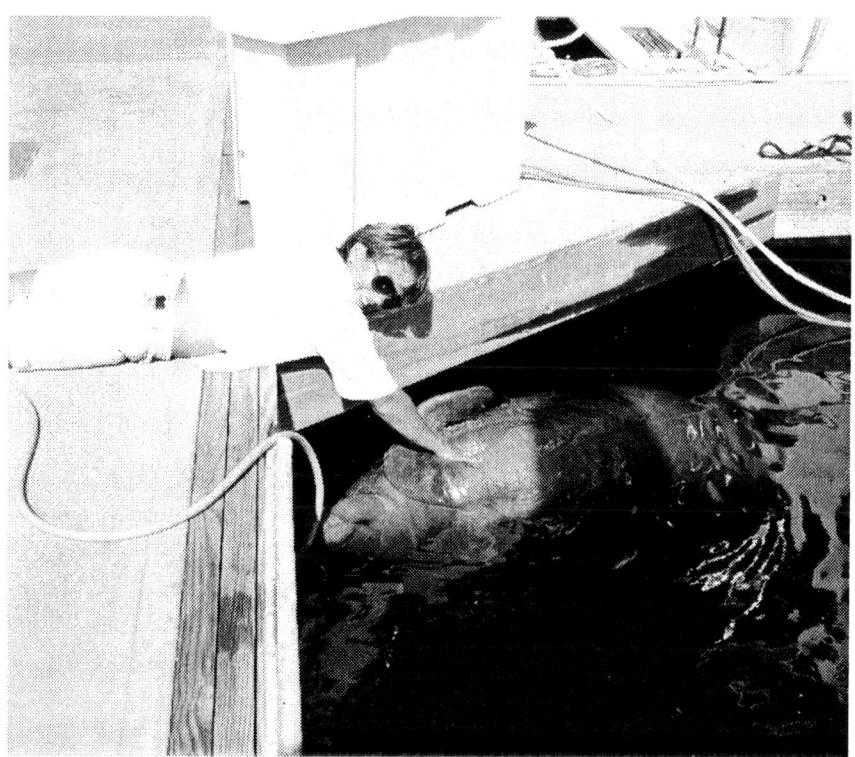

A manatee stops by for a belly rub at a marina in Florida.

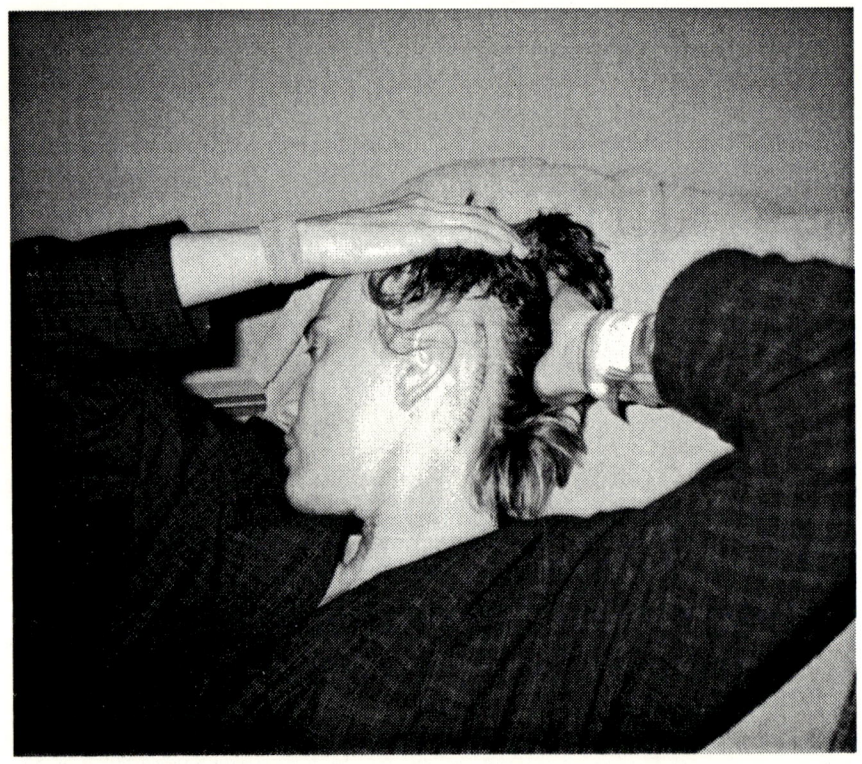

A souvenir from my bout with Trigeminal Neuralgia.

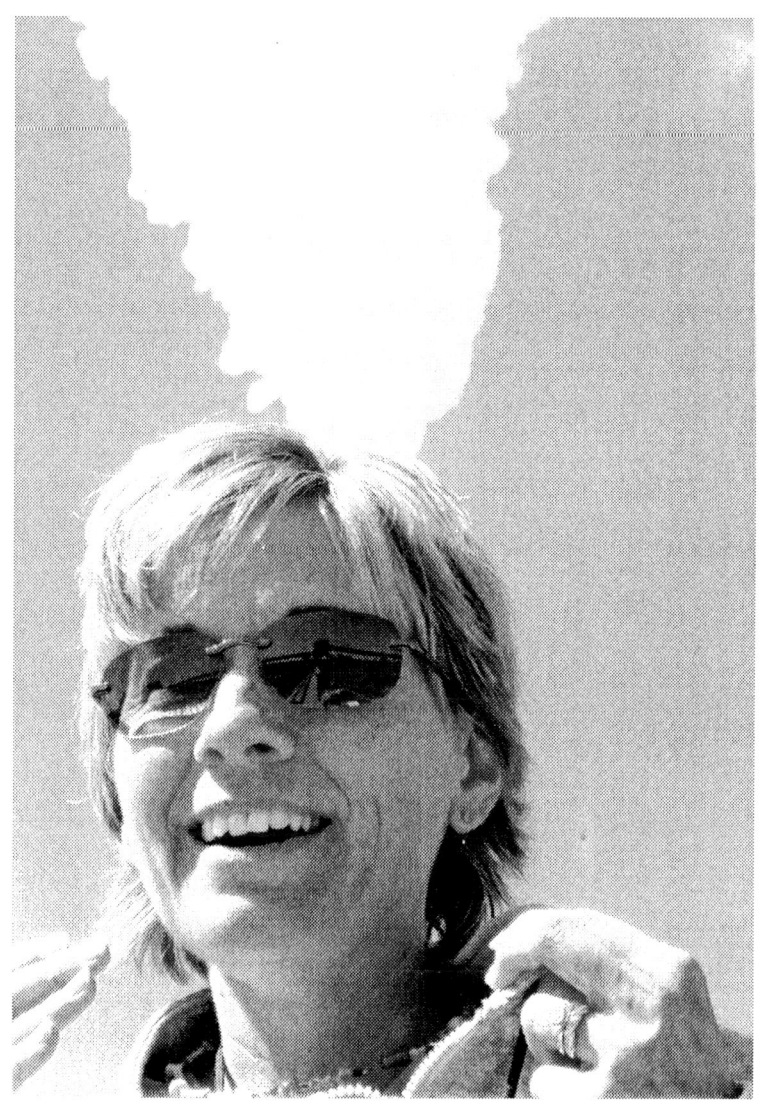

Pretending to have a hot flash.
(It's actually smoke from a power plant in the distance)

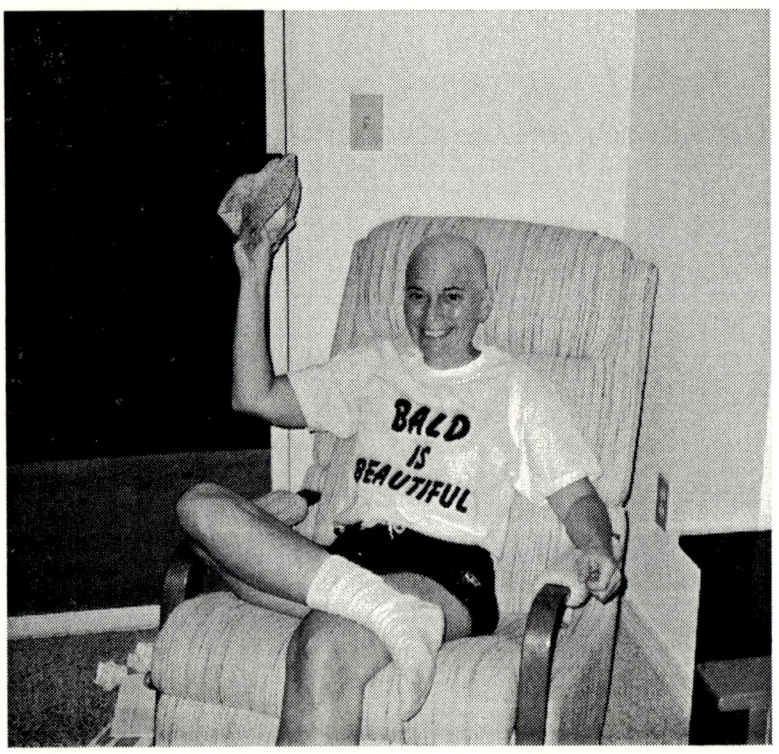

Showing off my hairless head.

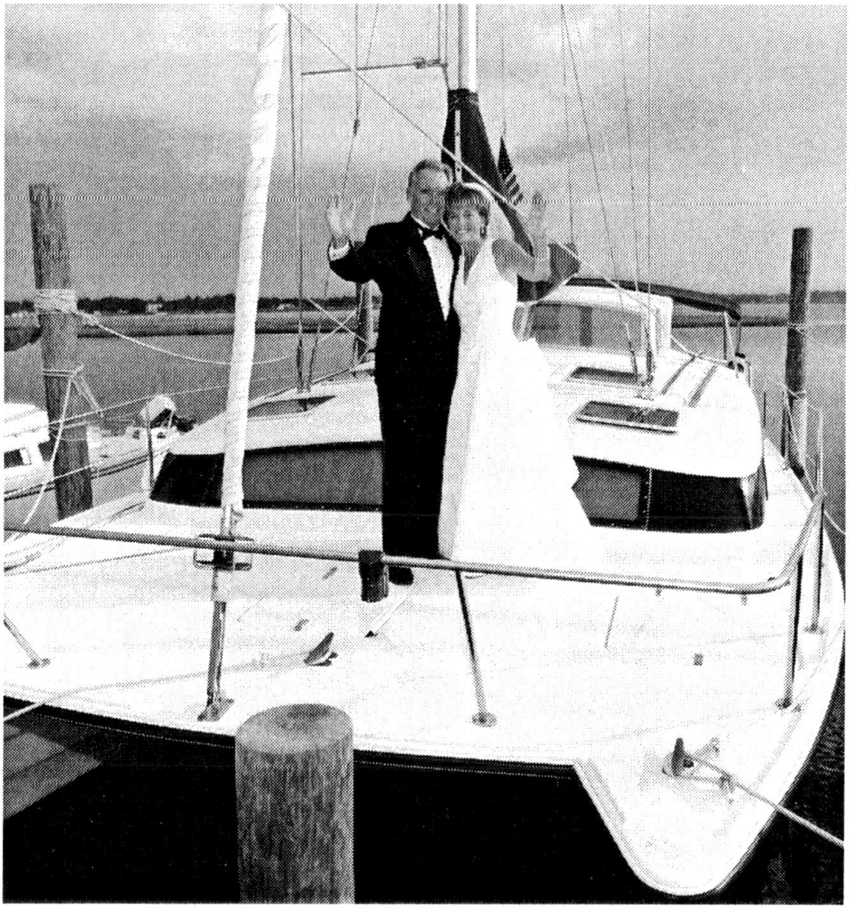

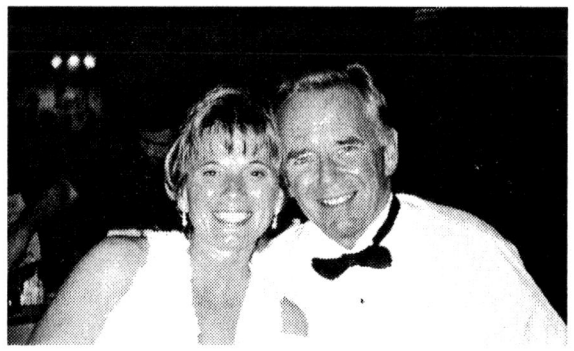

Our wedding day, September 25, 1999.

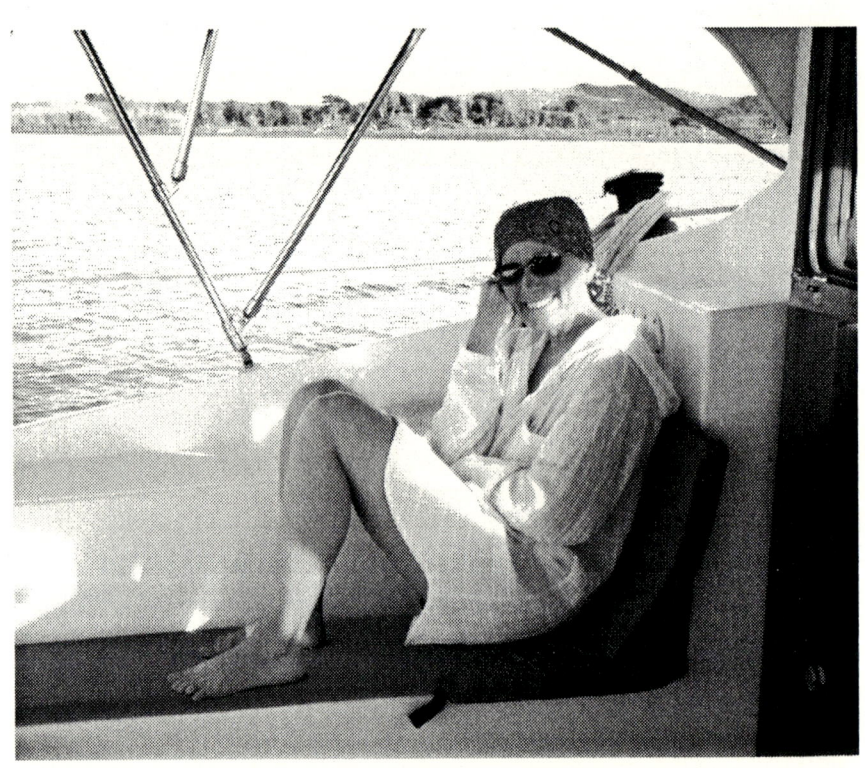

Relaxing aboard FREEDOM II.

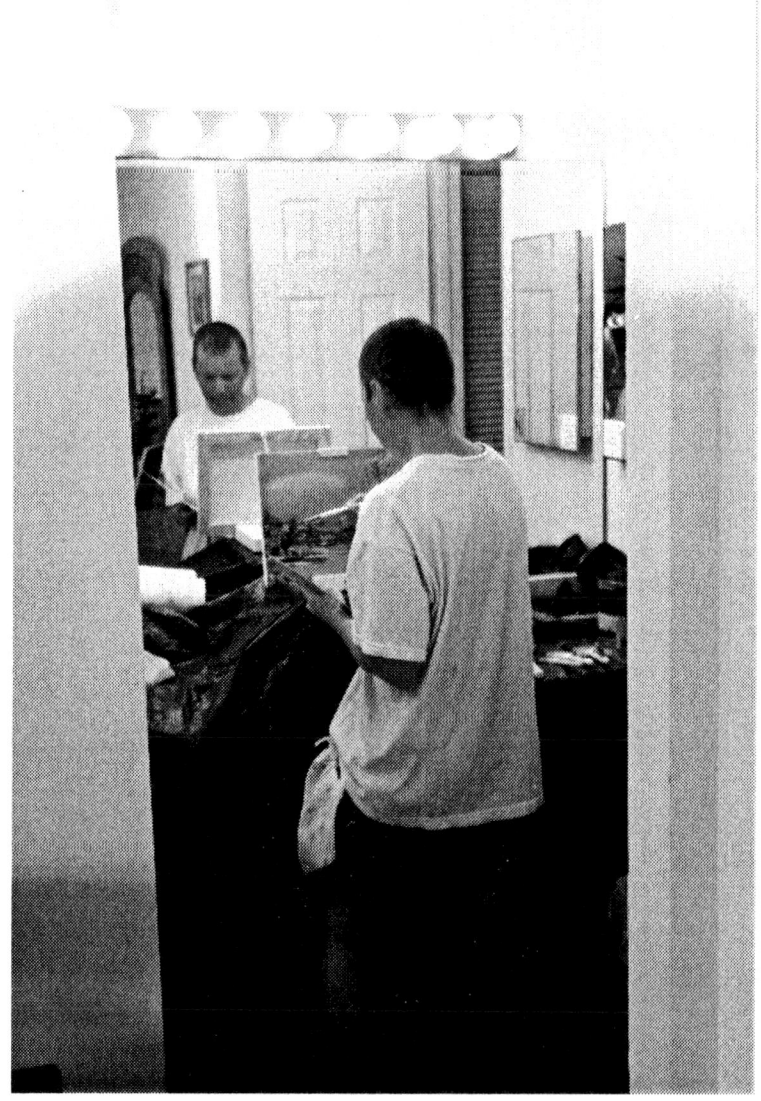

Trying my hand at a new hobby.
(My hair was starting to grow back
After taking a break from chemo.)

Part Two

%

My Story

"Preface"

People often ask, "How do you live with cancer?" as if it was an obnoxious roommate rather than a life-changing illness. My answer to that question is simple. You live with (and in spite of) cancer one day at a time. It is an unpredictable and frightening disease that doesn't knock gently at your door. When cancer enters your life, it tears the door down, barges in, and makes itself comfortable wherever it damn well pleases.

There are many books, pamphlets, and organizations that are available to help prepare for, and survive, a diagnosis of cancer. The truth is, this disease affects people in different ways. People with similar diagnoses may receive different treatments. People taking the same treatment may experience different side effects. Some people have a stronger support system than others. Each person needs to learn about their particular cancer, and what works best for him or her.

I learned a lot about how to deal with my cancer from a very unlikely source.

In 1992 I was given a unique opportunity. My boyfriend, Ed (who would later become my husband), asked me if I would like to live with him aboard his sailboat and cruise to the Florida Keys, the Bahamas and other destinations that offered sunshine, palm trees, and clear, tropical waters.

In order to do this I would have to sell, or give away, most of my "things", give up my apartment, put my car in storage, say goodbye to my family and friends, and quit my job as the director of one of the largest community-based drug and alcohol prevention, treatment, and education programs in the State of New York.

I know that there are thousands of people who would not hesitate to drop everything for the opportunity to sail over the horizon. I was not one of those people. I had never been on a boat for more than a couple of hours at a time. I knew absolutely nothing about living on a boat. I wasn't sure if I wanted to give up my current lifestyle for one filled with so much uncertainty.

In searching for the perfect word to describe my feelings about living on a sailboat and cruising to ports unknown, I looked up the word "frightened" in my thesaurus. There I found the synonyms dread, terror, alarm, panic, consternation, and fear. I then looked up the word "fear", and found the synonyms worry, anxiety, doubt, and dismay. In my continuing effort to find the perfect word to describe my feelings, I considered these: trepidation, jitters, creeps, cold sweat, nightmare, quivering, funk, and the ever popular, heebie-jeebies.

Not only did I have a difficult time defining my feelings, I had a difficult time prioritizing them as well.

What if I fall overboard? What if Ed falls overboard? What if a whale turns our boat over? How am I supposed to take a hot shower? What if I get claustrophobic? How will I do the laundry? What will we do about alligators, snakes, and sharks, coming near our boat? Where will I shop for food? How will we get our mail? What if I get seasick? What if one of us breaks a leg; has a heart attack; gets pneumonia; has the flu; worms; warts; hives; sunburn; bee sting? What if? Where? When? Why? Why? Why???

Ed had dreamed about sailing, scuba diving, and living on his own boat since he was a small child. My childhood in Brooklyn did not consist of boating, or scuba diving. A fun day in the water at my house meant that my parents had connected a small sprinkler to a garden hose in our cement backyard, and let my brother, my two sisters, and me take turns leaping through the water as it sprayed up at us. Some days, for variety, my mother or father would drape the hose through the basketball hoop that was attached to our garage, and we'd let the water rain down on us from above, rather than squirt up at us from below.

Ed went sailing. I played stoopball.

Ed went scuba diving. I played box baseball.

I was a Brooklyn girl. Water sports were not an important part of my life.

Needless to say, I was less than thrilled with the idea of changing my lifestyle to one that was unfamiliar, and frightening to me.

However, after months of soul-searching, I decided that I would join Ed on this journey.

Why? Was it a case of temporary insanity? Did I do it for love? Did I do it for the adventure? The challenge?

I guess it was all of the above. Mostly, I decided to follow this path in my life because I knew that if I didn't, I would spend the rest of my life wondering what I had missed. This was a once-in-a-lifetime offer. I would have to be crazy to not even allow myself to give it a try. The worst that could happen was that I would find it to be a miserable lifestyle, chalk it up to experience, and return to my old routine. The best that could happen was that I would find the courage to challenge myself, expand my life experiences, and see and do things that few people have the opportunity to be part of.

Ed bought a 32 ft. catamaran sailboat that he named FREEDOM II, after his last boat, FREEDOM. We moved on board in the summer of 1992. We lived aboard FREEDOM II for 5 full years, and we sailed her 21,000 miles. We sailed her from her homeport at the Timber Point marina on Long Island, New York to the coral reefs of the Florida Keys and the Bahamas.

I didn't fall in love with the lifestyle right away. I don't know when it happened, but somewhere along the journey I traded my anxiety for appreciation, my worry for wonder, and my fear for fun. That isn't to say that I had been transformed into Mrs. Ima Boater. I still had many moments when I couldn't relax for fear of what lay ahead. However, I found that most of the anxieties eased as I became more knowledgeable about the boat, about the water, and about my own abilities.

I became addicted to the excitement and the adventure of being one with nature. I loved watching the reflections on the water in the early mornings before any boats had a chance to ripple the surface. I cherished the peaceful calm at the end of a days run. I enjoyed sharing stories with other people who were out there, "doing it". It was a magical time filled with moonlit sails in the ocean; traveling the Intracoastal Waterway (ICW); spending time in nature, and visiting out of the way seaside villages.

Ed and I went swimming with dolphins. We pet manatees. We fell asleep to the distinct sounds of whippoorwills, wild boar, and alligators splashing their tails near the edge of the shore. We experienced the most spectacular, awe-inspiring displays of nature. We shared peaceful nights at anchor with friends who shared a common dream, a love of freedom, and a yearning for adventure.

As with many things in life, along with the good times, came some bad times. Our journey included battling terrifying storms, having boats (including our own) dragging anchor in the wee hours of the morning, and having our boat (our home) stolen. Drunks had crashed into our boat at two o'clock one morning; and we had a four-foot snake climb onto our boat in the middle of the night.

These "bad" experiences proved to be the very things that challenged us and helped us to grow as sailors, and as people.

Every day aboard FREEDOM II was a total immersion into the real world with circumstances that Ed and I had no control over, yet had to deal with. When a crisis occurred, there was no time to ask ourselves "Can we do this?" Or "Can we handle this?". We simply did what needed to be done, and in doing so we learned what we were made of.

Cruising under sail gave me confidence in myself. It taught me that I CAN handle life's challenges. The lessons that I learned while living and cruising aboard FREEDOM II were invaluable in preparing me for my battle against cancer. It taught me to slow down. I was used to a world of fast food, one-hour photos, microwaves, faxes, speed dialing, and express lanes. I needed to be moving, doing, going. I had no idea where I was going, or what I needed to do, but I was hell bent on getting there and doing it.

Cruising under sail taught me to slow down and enjoy the present moment.

Under sail or power, FREEDOM II would do an average of 6 knots. At this speed I had the pleasure of experiencing the world as it passed me by, or more accurately, as I passed by it.

I watched turtles sunning themselves on logs on the edge of the waterway. I smelled honeysuckle in the air and felt the cool breeze on my face. I heard the sound of dolphins breathing. I was able to experience cruising with all of my senses, touching it, smelling it, feeling it, and living it.

In the beginning, I found myself being envious of the power boaters who would reach anchorages hours, or even days ahead of us.
Once I challenged myself to ignore what the boaters around me were doing and concentrate on...experience...my present moment, I realized that there was little for me to envy.

I witnessed sights and sounds that they, racing through the waterway, could not possibly have noticed. Ed and I often watched as powerboats raced through a narrow strip of water coming within inches of hitting a manatee. Aside from the obvious danger of powering at such a high speed, they also missed watching this prehistoric creature floating so gracefully in it's natural environment. How many people in their lifetime will ever have that opportunity? What a shame it would have been to speed right by it.

Life with cancer literally takes the wind out of your sails. It makes you slow down. It is a life of waiting. Waiting for blood tests. Waiting for scans. Waiting for results. Waiting for the effects of the chemo to pass. Waiting to feel good. It's like being under sail in a world full of powerboats. The world races on, and some days you feel like you're not a part of it. I'm not sure how well I would have handled the waiting had it not been for my 5 years aboard FREEDOM II. I learned to have patience when dealing with forces that were beyond my control. I learned that I was able to handle more adversity than I ever could have imagined.

Cruising, like cancer, is a life of ups and downs. One day the sun is shining, the wind is a perfect 10-15 knots, and the current is pushing your vessel gently down the waterway. The next day it's raining, the wind kicks up to 35-40 knots, and the seas are turbulent and confused. Ed and I needed to be willing to adjust our sails, chart a different course, and change our destination. We had to know when it was prudent to seek safe harbor, anchor the boat, and wait for better weather.

Life with cancer is no different. It has good days and bad days. Some days I was filled with energy. I knew that those were the days to get chores done. Those were the days to do the laundry and the grocery shopping, get together with friends, and enjoy feeling good. Other days I needed to anchor myself, and wait out the storm. I needed to allow myself time to curl up on the couch, sleep, ask other people for help, and wait to feel better.

The most valuable lesson that cruising taught me about living with cancer, is that bad times, like good times, come and go. And, although the bad times are frightening, and painful to endure, they are there to help us learn and grow. The most terrifying days aboard FREEDOM II are the ones that I look back on with the most pride, because I know that I had courage, I remained strong, and I survived.

"Your Toothache Needs Brain Surgery"

January 16, 1997 marked the beginning of the end of our cruising aboard FREEDOM II.

That was the night that a mysterious medical condition entered my life. It wasn't cancer. It had nothing to do with the cancer that was still in my future. However both medical challenges shared much in common. In both instances I would work with doctors in New York and Florida. Initial tests for both proved to be inconclusive or incorrect. Both conditions would put me on a roller coaster of emotions as I searched for the proper diagnosis. It was almost as if this experience had been given to me as preparation for the fight of my life that was yet to come.

Ed and I were enjoying our fifth winter in Marathon, Florida in the fabulous Florida Keys. We were having dinner with some friends and fellow cruisers. All of a sudden I felt as if someone, or something had electrocuted the lower left side of my face. Like a flash of lightning, a sharp pain shot from my left ear into my lower jaw. As abruptly as it hit, the pain disappeared. The rest of the dinner passed without any further problems. I was relieved to know that it had just been a freak occurrence.

That night I woke from a deep sleep when an electrical shock bolted through my jaw. It lasted 3-5 seconds then subsided, only to "zap" me again moments later. The attacks continued on and off during the night. They came without warning, and left just as quickly.

I couldn't imagine what this mysterious pain could be, but I knew that I needed to get medical attention as soon as possible. Being live-aboard cruisers more than 1,000 miles from home, Ed and I did not have a car available to us. We would need to find a physician that we could walk to, ride bicycles to, or get to by boat.

Since the majority of the pain was in my lower jaw, I was convinced that I had a bad tooth that needed attention. I looked in the phone book, found the name of a local dentist, and made an appointment to see him.

The following morning we motored our dinghy through Boot Key Harbor, docked it by a cement pier, and walked one and a half miles to the dentist's office. After a quick examination he told me that I had an impacted wisdom tooth that may, or may not, be the source of the pain. He referred me to an oral surgeon, the nearest one being in Key West, 65 miles away.

Eight days later Ed and I rented a car and drove to the surgeon's office. After taking x-rays and giving me an examination, he agreed that I had an impacted wisdom tooth that may, or may not, be the source of my pain. The only way to eliminate it as the culprit would be to pull it out. Unfortunately, that's what we did.

The surgeon sent me home with instructions to keep cold compresses on my jaw to keep the swelling down. The compresses made the electrical shocks worse, so I decided to stop using them. My jaw swelled so badly that I couldn't open it at all. It locked shut. Even worse, the electric shocks continued. Obviously, the tooth had not been the problem.

The surgeon advised me to use moist heat to loosen the jaw muscles. The heat made the attacks come more often, and they were getting more severe. At one point it felt like fireworks were going off inside of my face. I stopped using the heat, and waited for the jaw to loosen on its own.

One week later, Ed and I rented another car and drove to the surgeon's office to have the stitches removed. I told him about the ongoing pain. He told me that I should seek other medical attention, as it did not appear to be a dental problem.

I took the phone book out again and located a general practitioner who was within walking distance of the marina. Ed and I walked three miles to the doctor's office hoping to find out what this strange condition was. By this time the pains were coming every day, and they would occur at least a dozen times a day.

I gave the doctor a description of the pains and told him about my experience with the dentist and the oral surgeon. After taking my medical history and giving me a physical examination, he said that he suspected either Lyme disease or Rheumatoid arthritis. He ordered blood to be drawn and tested. My follow-up appointment would be in four days.

I found myself praying that the doctor would find something wrong. I wanted a diagnosis so that a treatment could be started to take the pain away. But, after walking back to the doctor's office, I learned that I did not have Lyme disease, or Rheumatoid Arthritis. I asked the obvious question, "What do I have?" The doctor shrugged.

I suggested that there might be something wrong with my ear, since that's where the pains seemed to stem from. He checked my ear. It was fine. I suggested that my jaw might be out of alignment. I had dislocated my jaw as a teenager. I thought that these pains might somehow be connected. He checked my jaw. It, too, was fine. The doctor said it was "probably" just an inflammation. He gave me an anti-inflammatory shot and some pills, and told me to come back in one week.

The pains never let up. I would wake up during the night grabbing at my face. I would be talking on the telephone, and drop the receiver as I was hit with another flash of lightning. I would simply turn my head, and I'd get zapped.

I couldn't wait a whole week for my next appointment. The anti-inflammatory pills weren't doing anything to ease the pain. Ed suggested that I see a neurologist.

The neurologist took my medical history, checked my reflexes, and tested my eyes and coordination. Then he gave me horrible news. He announced that I was perfectly healthy. I could have cried. I didn't want to hear that I was perfectly healthy. Something was wrong with me, and no one was able to tell me what it was.

After another round of tests, and more waiting, the neurologist said it was possible that I had a condition called Trigeminal Neuralgia (TN). Having never heard of TN, I didn't know how to react to this news.

He told me that Trigeminal Neuralgia (also called Tic Doulourex, which means "painful spasm" in French) is a disorder of the fifth cranial nerve, the main nerve that supplies impulses from your face to your brain. He said that possible causes of the pain were: a blood vessel in the brain pressing on the trigeminal nerve; a tumor in the brain pressing on the nerve; or the onset of Multiple Sclerosis (MS).

He ordered an MRI of the brain. The results showed no signs of MS, no tumor, and no blood vessel pressing on the nerve. He said that the Trigeminal Nerve was just "damaged". He prescribed a medication called Tegretol, also known as Carbamezapine. Tegretol is an anticonvulsant that is usually prescribed for epileptics. It is believed that it can also be useful in easing the pain of TN.

Some of the side effects of Tegretol can include dizziness, lightheadedness, and disorientation. I told the doctor that Ed and I were beginning our cruise back to New York on FREEDOM II. I couldn't afford to be dizzy and disoriented on a boat at sea. He put me on a very low dose, 100 mgs, and told me that I would be able to increase it if needed. Ed and I knew that this trip home aboard FREEDOM II would be our last. We didn't know what the outcome of this condition would be, but we knew that it would be wise to stay closer to land, and closer to medical attention.

In early March, we left Marathon. It was a bittersweet trip home. Many times we stood in the cockpit and watched a favorite part of the waterway disappear over the horizon or around a bend. I was filled with incredible sadness, yet I also felt deep gratitude that I had seen so many wonderful things, met so many interesting people, and been so many exciting places.

My appreciation deepened with the realization that I would never be this way again. I would never again anchor in my favorite cove, dinghy through the mangroves, or watch dolphins swim beside my boat. I wanted to burn each sight, sound and smell into my memory to insure that they would never be forgotten. I realized how much I had taken for granted over the past 5 years.

That final journey home aboard FREEDOM II, helped me understand the importance of grabbing onto life, and making the most of every moment. I learned to stop taking things for granted. I learned to appreciate people, places, and things, because I can never know when they might be taken from me. I learned that the journey might be shorter than I think.

Within days of arriving home I saw my primary care physician. He referred me to a neurologist for further tests. The neurologist told me that there still was a possibility that I was experiencing the onset of MS. Once again my heart sank. I was learning quickly that there is no definitive test for the existence of TN.

After two more MRI's, I was told that there was no sign of a tumor or MS. It was assumed that I had a blood vessel that was pulsing on the Trigeminal nerve, wearing through the myelin lining. The vessel would not show up on any of the tests. It was only by the process of elimination, and by my description of the pains, that this diagnosis was made.

I was referred to a neurosurgeon in New York City who agreed with the diagnosis of TN. He increased the Tegretol to 400 mgs per day. The pains continued. He increased it again. This time to 600 mgs. I felt drowsy a great deal of the time which, I knew, was to be expected.

From the moment that I heard the words Trigeminal Neuralgia, I became an information junkie. I wanted to know everything there was to know about this condition, about brain tumors, and about Multiple Sclerosis. Mostly I wanted to investigate all of the possible treatments and/or cures.

It wasn't until I read an article on Trigeminal Neuralgia that I realized how lucky I was to have been diagnosed so quickly. I read about one woman who had 23 root canals before she was correctly diagnosed. Another woman had been suffering with the pain for ten years before she was diagnosed. Still another sufferer had had all of her teeth pulled before she was properly diagnosed. I read that TN received the nickname "The Suicide Disease". The unrelenting pain, along with the lack of a clear diagnosis, had so overwhelmed some victims of TN that they had taken their own lives.

I read, I researched, and I asked a lot of questions. After meeting with the neurosurgeon two more times it was decided that the medication was not working. I had the option to further increase the dosage, or to have surgery. I did not like the effects of the medication. I felt disoriented and drowsy most of the time. Surgery offered me a good chance of being pain free, and medicine free, for the rest of my life. That's what I chose to do.

The procedure, called microvascular decompression (MVD), is the most invasive of all the procedures for TN, but it offered the most permanent solution in my case. Unfortunately, none of the procedures for Trigeminal Neuralgia are 100% effective in all cases.

MVD surgery involves shaving behind the ear on the affected side, and making an incision approximately 4 1/2 inches in length. A hole, approximately the size of a half dollar is made in the skull, the trigeminal nerve is viewed through an operating microscope and any compressing blood vessels are lifted off of the nerve. The nerve is then protected with a soft pad usually made of shredded teflon.

The surgery was a success. The surgeon told me that he had found a vessel that was actually knuckled, or bent right into the nerve, and that had been the source of my pain. I was relieved. I was also relieved to notice that the pain was completely gone, (and it has never returned).

After months of stiffness, headaches, nausea, soreness, and difficulty hearing out of my left ear, I made a full recovery. Ed and I decided that if we couldn't be snowbirds on the water, we would be snowbirds on land. We kept FREEDOM II as a summer home in New York, and rented a townhouse in Jensen Beach, Florida for the winters.

We greatly missed being full time, live-aboard cruisers, but spending six months in Florida, and living on the boat on Long Island for the other six months of the year was a good compromise.

Winters in Florida allowed us to continue spending the majority of our time outdoors. We went for walks along the ocean, rented canoes, and made good use of the swimming pool, which was only 100 steps from our front door. We spent our summers sailing, going to the ocean, and enjoying time with family and friends. Before long Ed and I adjusted to our new life. We knew that we would always miss cruising, but we also knew that we had nothing to complain about. We were retired. We were having fun. And we were both healthy.

Little did we know, all of that was about to change.

"It's Nothing To Worry About"

One morning in February 2002, while showering after a relaxing swim in the pool, I found a lump in my right breast. This large, oval-shaped lump had not been there in January. I was sure of that. It seemed to have appeared overnight.

I immediately ran downstairs to Ed, and had him feel it. There was no missing this huge, lumpy mass. It was approximately 2 inches long and 1 inch wide. We remained calm, took out our health insurance book and started to look for a doctor in our area.

It was our third winter in Jensen Beach. Neither of us had the need for a doctor until now, so I didn't know who to call. I looked in my insurance company's provider directory, and found a physician who was on our plan. Luckily, she was only 10 minutes away. I called her office, and was given an appointment for the following day.

The physician felt the lump, told me that it could just be fibrous tissue, but that she would send me for a mammogram to have it checked out. I had been going for yearly mammograms for the past seven years, starting when I was 35 years old. I was all too familiar with the pulling, squishing, flattening routine.

Perhaps the only thing that is more uncomfortable than the pulling, squishing, and flattening, is the agony of waiting for the results.

A few days after the exam I received a call from the doctor's office telling me that the results of the mammogram were negative.

"What do you mean the results are negative?" I asked, relieved yet confused.

"It means that the test was normal."

"Then what is this huge lump in my breast?"

"I don't know," The voice on the other end said, "The report just says that the results are normal."

"There's nothing normal about having a huge lump in my breast. I need to know what it is."

The voice told me that she would check with my doctor and get back to me. She did.

"You have fibrocystic breast disease." She explained. "The lump is just thick fibrous tissue. It's nothing to worry about."

Maybe it's just me, but anytime I hear the word "disease" attached to a condition that's in my body, I tend to worry. I told this to the nurse, who was rapidly losing her patience with me.

"It isn't actually a disease," She explained, "it's just a condition that means you have thick tissue in your breast. Many women have it. It's nothing to worry about."

There were those five beautiful words again...'It's nothing to worry about.' Those were exactly the words I was hoping to hear.

The doctor recommended a yearly check-up, and nothing more.

I was relieved, to say the least.

Ed and I spent the rest of the winter and the following summer doing what we do best, relaxing and enjoying life. We took long walks on the beaches. We sailed as often as the weather would allow. We went to backyard barbeques; we visited friends and family, and invited them to spend time with us aboard FREEDOM II.

On September 3, I had an appointment with my gynecologist in New York for a pap smear and a check up. The GYN felt the lump in my breast.

"That's nothing." I assured him. "I had it checked out already, it's just fibrous tissue."

I have known this GYN for many years. I know when he is happy with what he is feeling and when he isn't. Unfortunately, this time he was not.

"This isn't 'nothing'." He said.

He referred me to a breast specialist and to a lab for another mammogram.

I wasn't worried. I knew that this was routine, and that the G-Y-N had to cover his you-know-what. After all, I was living in an area with one of the highest rates of breast cancer in the country. I appreciated how cautious and thorough he was being.

I scheduled the mammogram with the lab, and made the appointment with the specialist.

The day before the mammogram, I participated in a walk-a-thon for autism. My niece, Katie and I walked three miles at a pretty fast pace. I felt energized, alive and extremely healthy. In fact, the walk felt so good that I asked Katie if she wanted to make it a weekly thing. I was convinced more than ever that the lump in my breast was "nothing to worry about". I simply felt too good to be sick.

I went to the lab feeling happy and optimistic. After more pulling, squishing, and flattening, the lab technician left the room to make sure that the films were "readable". When she came back into the room, she told me that something didn't seem right. They wanted me to have another test done on the right breast. This time it would be a sonogram.

I would have to wait until my appointment with the breast specialist to get the results of both of these tests.

Ed offered to come with me to see the surgeon. I was confident that it was going to be a simple and quick exam. I told him that I would go by myself.

The surgeon felt the lump in my right breast and without hesitation said, "This needs to come out." He showed me the films from the mammogram. They showed nothing. The sonogram, however, did show a large mass in the upper, inner quadrant of my breast. "Are we talking about cancer?" I asked. My heart and my stomach were now competing for room in my throat. I wished that I had taken Ed up on his offer to come with me. "I can't tell right now. It's probably benign, but we can't be sure. It needs to come out so we can test it."

He explained that the lump was too large for a needle biopsy. It would be too easy to hit a "healthy" spot and miss a "diseased" spot in a lump that was so large. The only way to test it would be to take the entire lump out. He said that he could schedule me for surgery on Friday. Only four days away.

I was stunned. Things were moving so fast. I agreed to the date, only because I didn't know what else to do. I said, "I'm sure I should be asking you a ton of questions right now, but I have no idea what to ask."

The surgeon gave me all the information that he thought I needed. How long of an operation it would be, what the incision would look like, how long I'd be in the hospital, and so on. Half of what he said went in one ear and out the other. I didn't hear a word he said beyond, "this needs to come out".

I tend to be an optimist at heart. I always believe that good things will happen even in the darkest moments. Even now, I was willing to bet money that all I had was a benign lump that would be removed and life would go on as usual.

Along with my optimism comes a healthy skepticism of people who want to make deep gashes in my body in order to remove parts of me that I've grown to know and love. I decided to cancel the surgery scheduled for that Friday and give myself time to go for a second opinion, and a third if need be.

The second doctor agreed that the mass was probably benign but should be removed and tested. He seemed to think that it was not likely to be cancer because of the way it had popped up so suddenly. Ed and I left his office feeling good about what he had said. When I got home, I called the first doctor back and scheduled the surgery for his next available date. It was only two weeks away.

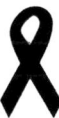

"It Is Cancer"

I had no fear going into the surgery. As a matter of fact I was joking around quite a bit. I had had 2 mammograms that came back clear. I had the doctor in Florida who told me that it was nothing to worry about. I had two additional doctors agree that it was probably benign, but it needed to come out to be tested. I NEVER entertained the thought that it could be cancer...NEVER.

Ed and my mother came to the hospital with me. I changed into a very "stylish" hospital gown with matching hat and booties. The nurses came in to hook me up to an IV bag, and then proceeded to ask me a ton of questions.

As they wheeled me into the operating room, I smiled at Ed and my mother, gave them each a kiss and said, "Don't worry." I hated the look of fear in their eyes. After all, this was just a benign lump that was going to be taken out. Everything would be fine.

I woke up in the recovery room. Hours had passed. I started to throw up, which is what I tend to do after being given anesthesia...on an empty stomach…early in the morning…after having a team of people cut into my body. No surprise there!

The surgeon woke me from my precious sleep. "We got the lump out." He said, then added, "It IS cancer." Maybe it was the anesthesia, maybe it was the painkillers, or maybe it was my mind's ability to deny what it had just heard, but I felt no emotion at all. He may as well have just informed me that it's raining outside. I just looked at him with no emotion and said, "It is?"

He nodded.

My mother and my husband were in the waiting area. My first concern was for them.

"Did you tell Ed and my mother?"

Another nod.

"How did they take it?"

"Not as well as you are."

(Three cheers for being numbed by drugs.)

I don't remember anything else until I found myself in a different room. I opened my eyes to see my husband walking…staggering towards me. He was shaking like a leaf.

"Did the doctor tell you?" He asked.

My turn to nod.

He broke down and cried. I wanted to cry with him, but I was too numb. I had no tears. I had no fear of this disease that had entered my life. I know now that my lack of fear was ignorance of what was to come.

My mother came in a while later. I didn't know what to say to her. I'm sure that she was at a loss for words herself.

"I'm just full of surprises, aren't I?" I said.

Ed told me that after hearing the news from the surgeon, he and my mother held each other and cried. I saw that my mother's eyes were swollen and red, but she seemed to be handling it pretty well for my sake.

I don't remember much of their visit. I drifted in and out of sleep for quite some time. My mother left for home to start the difficult task of spreading the news to my family.

Hours later Ed and I went home. (You don't stay in the hospital overnight for such a "minor" procedure.)

Neither of us spoke on the car ride home. I needed to sit quietly and digest all that was happening to me. Ed respected my need for privacy. I'm sure he was trying to figure out how to deal with the turmoil in his own mind.

When we arrived home I took two pain pills and went to sleep. Ed joined my parents in making and answering phone calls. Many people knew that I had been scheduled for surgery that day. They all asked to be "kept in the loop" via telephone or e-mail. I knew that it couldn't be easy for Ed or my parents to repeat the story over and over again, but they were great about doing it.

My parents called my siblings and dozens of family friends, asking them to spread the news. Ed called his daughter Amy, and his sister Marcia, asking them to do the same. Reactions ranged from sadness, to anger, to stunned silence. Many people asked if it would be all right for them to come for a visit. I wasn't ready for that. I wasn't sure when I would be.

"Help Me Feel Normal Again"

My breast was bandaged from the middle of my rib cage to under my armpit, and from just below my shoulder to the bottom of my ribs. It seemed like an enormous amount of gauze and tape, and it made me wonder just how big the incision was. Any scar on your body is upsetting. A scar on the breast is even more so. The breast is the place where we nurture children. It is a part of our sexuality. It is a part of our femininity.

I knew that one of the most frightening moments would be taking the bandage off to see what the breast looked like underneath. That would happen the following day.

In the meantime, I napped on and off. My parents and Ed were bombarded with phone calls from friends and family who had heard the news. These phone calls continued for days, then days turned into weeks. Ed and I could not sit down to a half-hour TV show and watch it straight through without the phone interrupting us. Lunch and dinner were spent half eating, half talking on the phone. The support and love that we received was overwhelming. The outpouring of prayers and good wishes lifted our spirits at a time when we needed it most. Although I felt desperate for rest, I did not want to miss a single call. Hearing the love in the voices of close friends and family helped both of us get through those first couple of weeks with our sanity intact.

The phone calls reminded us that we were not alone. They helped us to focus on the number of friends that we have and the support system that is available to us. The phone calls helped us to maintain a piece of normalcy in our lives at a time when everything seemed to be falling apart.

At one point, my younger sister, Grace, asked, "What do you want my role in this to be?" I told her that, as much as possible, I just wanted her to help me feel normal again.

My whole life I have relied on my sense of humor to help me deal with difficult circumstances. I have always been the sister who made jokes all the time. I was the kid with the witty comeback who loved to laugh. I was the aunt who would drop down to the floor to wrestle with my nieces and nephews, give them piggyback rides and play make-believe games. Literally overnight all of that changed. Friends who used to e-mail me jokes, only sent e-mails offering prayers. Others wouldn't call because they didn't know what to say. Still others would call and talk in hushed tones. Family members who used to engage in playful teasing with me, no longer dared to tease. I couldn't play with my nieces and nephews because I was too sore from the surgery. On the rare occasions when I would joke and make light of the situation, I could feel the discomfort in those around me, so I stopped joking. I knew that my sister, who has also been my best friend throughout my life, would understand what I meant by "help me feel normal again."

It was an emotionally confusing time for me on many levels. I didn't want cancer to monopolize all of my conversations. Yet, it felt awkward to talk with my friends and not mention it at all. My relationships turned into a delicate dance of protecting feelings, avoiding certain emotions and trying to maintain a piece of the "old me". I knew that it would all become more comfortable over time, but that did nothing to ease my frustration. After all, who wants cancer to become part of their comfort zone?

Taking off the bandage was physically and emotionally painful. Physically it hurt like a son-of-a-gun because of all the tape that had been used to adhere it to the skin. Between losing some of the breast, throwing up, and leaving a great deal of my skin on hospital gauze and tape, I was sure that I had lost at least 10 pounds.

I went in the bathroom alone. I wanted to be the first one to see what my breast (or lack of breast) looked like. I faced away from the mirror as I took off the bulky dressing. I was afraid to see the incision. I was afraid to see how much of my breast had been removed. I didn't look down at myself for quite some time.

Many thoughts went through my mind. One of those thoughts was of Ed. How would he react when he saw what my breast looked like? I was confident that his reaction should be the least of my worries. I knew that Ed would support me and love me no matter what I looked like. Our relationship had been tested over and over again during our cruising years. There was no challenge that we hadn't faced together. Each challenge brought us closer together. We were always there to support one another through the good times and the bad. I knew that he would continue to be a great source of strength, love and support for me. Still, I was nervous and afraid.

With the dressing off I, oh-so-slowly turned my body toward the mirror.

I looked at myself for the first time and almost cried.

I almost screamed.

Maybe I did scream.

"I have a 90 year old boob!!!"

My breast, what was left of it, was horribly wrinkled. It looked like the breast of a 90-year-old woman. (Not that I've seen many 90-year-old women naked, but you get the point.)

Somehow, I summoned the nerve to take a closer look. I am thankful that I did. What I hadn't realized was that underneath all of the bandages, the incision was still covered with clear tape. The tape was pulling at the skin, causing it to look wrinkled. I sat down with a huge sigh of relief.

This clear tape would stay on until my next doctor's appointment.

The incision turned out to be 4 inches long going from the top of the areola upwards. It was red and swollen and ugly, but I knew that it would get better in time.

I couldn't take a shower for a few days. When I finally did, I had to keep my back to the water. I got myself into some pretty "interesting" positions as I tried to wash my hair and body without getting any water on the clear tape that was left over the incision. I used clear wrap as an extra covering to keep the water away from the breast.

It seemed to take forever to make any progress in the mornings. I moved slower than usual. My showers took longer than usual. Drying my hair became a chore, and getting dressed became a long and painful process. I was only able to use one arm. My right arm was sore and stiff. I knew that I shouldn't baby it, but that's exactly what I wanted to do. I wanted to lie on the couch, lose myself in comedy shows on TV, laugh, and forget that I had been diagnosed with a life-threatening disease.

It wasn't going to be that easy.

"Whatever You Have, We Have"

On October 11th Ed and I drove to the surgeon's office to learn exactly what we were dealing with. This was quite possibly the longest ride of my life. I had no idea what kind of news I was about to receive, and I didn't know how to prepare myself.

I remembered back five years when Ed and I arrived at the neurologist's office to learn if I had MS, a tumor, or a malfunctioning blood vessel in my brain. Before going in the doctor's office, Ed stopped me, gave me a reassuring hug and said, "Whatever <u>you</u> have, <u>we</u> have."

I felt his love and support so strongly that day. I knew that no matter what happened, he would be there to help me through it.

As Ed and I drove to the breast surgeon's office that cold, October day, he took my hand and gently reminded me, "Remember, whatever <u>you</u> have, <u>we</u> have."

The surgeon told us that the cancer was at least stage II. He used terms like, clear margins, and invasive ductal carcinoma. He explained what these terms meant, and I was hoping that Ed was understanding it better than I was.

The surgeon told us that I had a marker that was elevated. There is a blood test, a cancer marker, called a CA 27.29   If it is elevated; it suggests that there could be cancer somewhere else in the body. A normal reading for this marker would be 0-38. Mine was 54. This put up a red flag that there could be more cancer somewhere.

It was a surreal experience sitting in that chair knowing that it was my body that was being talked about, yet feeling as if this horrible reality had nothing to do with me at all. I wanted so badly to remove myself from the situation, yet I knew that no matter where I went, IT would come with me. There would be no hiding, no running away, no pretending that everything was normal. Dealing with cancer would have to become my "new normal".

I also learned that I had tested negative for a gene called HER-2/neu. This is a gene that produces a receptor that helps cancer cells to grow. Testing negative was positive. It meant that I did not have the gene that tells the cancer cells to grow-grow-grow!

He said that my tumor was estrogen positive, which meant that the cancer cells were feeding off of the estrogen in my body. If it came down to it, we could shut off the estrogen and starve the cells of the food they need to live. This meant that I would go into chemically induced m-m-m-menopause. I have always feared menopause, and all that I've heard comes with it. Ed and I have a 20-year age difference. He used to joke that the only reason he married a younger woman was because with any luck, by the time I reached menopause, he'd be dead. It was starting to look like that might not be the case.

The surgeon told us that I would need to have another surgery to take some lymph nodes out of my armpit and check them for cancer.

He explained all of the particulars to us and we left his office in a daze of mixed emotions and medical jargon.

When we got home, Ed and I sat at the dining room table with my mother and father. We filled them in on everything that the doctor had said. We wanted to celebrate the fact that the tumor was gone, but the elevated marker was hanging over our heads. We tried to remain hopeful that the marker was high because the blood test had been taken <u>before</u> the tumor was removed. It made sense to us that with the cancerous mass out of the breast, the number would go back to normal. We would have to wait to find out if it had.

Ed and my parents took turns answering the phone, filling everyone in on the news. I appreciated having so many people call, but I wasn't ready to talk to anyone just yet. It seemed that all I talked about, read about or thought about anymore was cancer. I didn't want to talk about it for another second. I wanted to sit on the couch, watch a movie and lose myself in fantasy for a while.

"My 2nd (And 3rd) Surgeries"

The surgery was scheduled for October 25th. For this one I would stay in the hospital overnight. The surgeon had explained that after taking out and checking the lymph nodes, a drain would be inserted into my side, just below the incision. This drain would take out accumulated lymph fluid at the wound site.

He said that for approximately four days following the surgery, I would have a nurse come to the house to make sure that the drain was working properly. She would check my pulse, take my temperature, and make sure the wounds were healing as they should.

The night before the surgery I was surprisingly calm. I just wanted to get it over with. I didn't want to think about it anymore. I didn't want to worry about it anymore. I had gone for a second and third opinion before deciding to go ahead with the surgery. The decision was not whether or not to have the operation. It had to be done, that was a given. I needed to decide which procedure to go with. The procedure that I was scheduled for was called an axillary node dissection. That is when the surgeon removes a wad of fat from the hollow of the armpit, the axilla, which contains many of the lymph nodes. This tissue is sent to the pathologist, who examines the fat to see how may lymph nodes he can find and remove. The lymph nodes are tested to see if there is any cancer in them.

We had learned of another procedure called a sentinel node biopsy where, through the use of a blue dye or a radioactive tracer, the surgeon can find the one or two nodes that would most likely have cancer, and check them. This procedure allows for the removal of fewer lymph nodes, no drain is necessary, and there is less of a chance of lymphedema.

Lymphedema is an uncomfortable and sometimes severe and painful swelling of the arm. Once the lymph nodes are removed from underneath the armpit, the immune system to that arm is compromised. Any cut, burn, bug bite, sting or infection could bring on the condition, which there is no cure for. I had read that lymphedema is a life-long threat that could happen immediately following surgery or as much as twenty years later. (Apparently, just having cancer isn't enough of a challenge in and of itself.)

After meeting with various doctors we conducted our own research. We learned that if, during the sentinel node biopsy, a lymph node tested positive for cancer, a full axillary node dissection would have to be done anyway. That, plus the fact that the sentinel node biopsy was a relatively new procedure which had yet to be perfected, caused us to choose the tried and true dissection.

The night before the surgery I received a call from the surgeon. He had some news. The CA 27.29, which I had been tested for again, had gone down to 43. Going down was good, yet it was still elevated. The fact that the number was still outside of the normal range was not good news, but that wasn't the reason he was calling.

He said that after re-checking the slides of my original tumor, the pathologist found a microscopic spot in the margin. This meant that the margins were not as clear as they thought at first. When the surgeon removes a tumor, he takes some healthy tissue along with it. The section of healthy tissue makes up the margin. (I think of it as a piece of fruit with a rotten section taken out of it. Usually, you take out the rotten section with a chunk of "healthy" fruit around it just to be sure that you got all of the "diseased" part out. Sometimes you miss a piece of diseased fruit within the healthy area.) That's what happened in my case.

My clear margin turned out to not be so clear after all. He informed me that he would have to open the breast up again to get more tissue out. I had been somewhat satisfied with how the breast looked after the first surgery. It wasn't great, but it wasn't too deformed. Now, they would have to open it up again, and remove even more of it.

The following morning I would have two surgeries instead of one. I had just started healing from the first surgery; this would be a severe set back. I had no tears. I had no anger. I just had a strange feeling of nothingness. I knew that getting angry at the surgeon, or at the pathologist, or at the world, would do me no good. I resigned myself to what needed to be done. I went to bed early and prayed for God to watch over me the following morning.

"Bed Pan Blues"

On October 25, 2002 I had the lymph nodes removed, the drain put in, and the breast opened up again. I was not quite as jovial going into this surgery as I had been the last one. Yet, in my never-ending optimism, I was convinced that the cancer had all been removed with the first operation and that the tests on the lymph nodes would come back negative.

When I opened my eyes after the surgery, the first thing that I did was throw up. (Anesthesia simply does not agree with me.) The second thing that I did was look at my right arm to see if it was swollen. I was so afraid of getting lymphedema. I checked my arm and my hand for any signs of swelling. I didn't see any.

I was in recovery for 3 hours before I was able to see my husband and my older sister, Loretta, who had accompanied him on this trip. They had been there for a total of 6 hours, waiting…just waiting. For me the surgery was easy, I slept. That part of the ordeal is always harder for the people who are waiting and worrying. I know. I've been on that end of it too.

After saying a brief hello to Ed and my sister, I asked for a shot for the pain. Immediately after it was administered, I looked at my exhausted visitors, smiled and said, "Wow, this is good". I told them that they might as well go home because I couldn't keep my eyes open. All I wanted to do was sleep.

Anyone who has had the unfortunate experience of being in a hospital for any length of time knows that it is the worst place to get any rest. Nurses come and go at all hours to take your temperature, check your blood pressure, and give you medication that is supposed to help you sleep. Of course, if they had stopped waking me up to take my temperature, check my blood pressure and give me medication, I would have slept just fine. I understand, of course, that they have a job to do and it is all in my best interest.

It didn't take long for me to find out that one of the most difficult things to do as a patient in a hospital is go to the bathroom. In order to avoid using the dreaded bedpan, I had to get out of bed and make it all the way to the bathroom while connected to an IV pole whose wheels fought me every step of the way. It would have been easier to use the bedpan...or would it?

What sadistic person invented the bedpan anyway? Is it just me, or does the pee always wind up leaking out the side, or the back of the pan? Is it, in fact, possible to situate a human heiny comfortably and conveniently on a pan of that shape without spillage? I tried sitting firmly on the pan, hovering over the pan, laying down on the pan, and sitting at an incline while holding on to the pan. It was no use. No matter how I approached it, I always had spillage. My predicament would have made a funny comedy routine if it hadn't been so humiliating.

Hospitals, I learned, are also the worst places to eat or drink. It was about 3:00 in the morning and I was dying of thirst. I attempted to reach the bottle of ginger ale that was sitting on the tray beside my bed. The surgery had been on my <u>right</u> side. The food tray had been placed on my <u>right</u> side. There was no way for me to reach it with my <u>right</u> hand. I attempted to reach over myself with my left hand, but it was a futile attempt. No matter how hard I tried, I couldn't reach the tray. I stared at the ginger ale and decided to call for help. I knew that there had to be a buzzer somewhere nearby that would allow me to alert the nurses to my need for assistance. After a quick search I saw the buzzer. It was on the bed, up by my <u>right</u> shoulder, just out of my reach. I gave up and went to sleep.

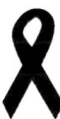

"The Cancer Has Spread"

It was October 31st, Halloween. Ed drove me to the surgeon's office to get the results of the lymph node surgery. Every bump in the road…and I mean EVERY bump in the road made the breast (what was left of it) pull on the incision, the staples, and the drain. I had to keep my hand inside of my shirt for the entire ride, gently holding onto my breast in an attempt to keep it from jiggling. I knew that other motorists had to wonder what cheap thrill I was getting with my hand inside of my shirt, but I really didn't care what they thought. All I knew was that my poor, deformed boob felt loved and supported for the first time in a long time. That's all that I cared about.

The surgeon told us that he had removed twelve lymph nodes. Two of them tested positive for cancer. I had myself convinced that all of the cancer had been taken out with the large tumor. This news hit me like a sledgehammer. The cancer had spread to the lymph nodes.

He also informed us that the cancer marker was still elevated. I would have to go for a series of tests to determine if there was more cancer, and if so, where. He told me that I would be scheduled for a bone scan and a CT scan of the chest, abdomen, and pelvis.

It seems that when breast cancer cells metastasize (spread) they usually go to the brain, the bone, the liver, or the lungs. What's so special about those areas is beyond me, but that's where they go. It was time for more tests.

I called the lab and scheduled the scans for the following week. In the meantime, my poor husband had the unpleasant job of cleaning my drain of "lymph juice" twice a day, and keeping a journal of how much juice came out each time. He was a real champ about it. I could not have imagined him being any more supportive than he was. I knew that this trauma that had entered our lives had to be getting to him too. Yet he remained strong for me. He kept his sense of humor. He encouraged me. And most importantly, he listened to me when I needed to talk.

One of the most important things that I had to do after the surgery was exercise my arm. After any surgery, your body's instinct is to protect the injury. I wanted to keep my arm pinned to my side where it was most comfortable. Unfortunately, this was the worst thing I could do. I was told to keep moving it. I had to literally climb the walls, inching my hands higher and higher up the wall, trying to reach further each day. Some days were better than others.

In the evenings my arm would be loose, and I would feel that I was making a great deal of progress. Things would stiffen up overnight, and the following morning I would not be able to reach as high as I had the previous day. It was infuriating. Ed was great at keeping me focused on the positive, and gently encouraged me along. He stood by me through my frustration, and he celebrated each victory with me

I had to squeeze a soft ball so that I would not lose strength in my hand. I also had a variety of exercises that I needed to do in order to keep flexibility and mobility in my shoulder.

A nurse came to the house each day to check my pulse, temperature and blood pressure. She checked the drain to make sure that it was working properly. She advised me to wear slippers with a non-skid bottom, and to keep moving my arm.

I wanted to do nothing but rest. However, between phone calls, having visitors, reading about cancer, and doing my exercises, cancer became a full time job. I loved the phone calls and the visits. They helped to cheer me up and kept my mind off of my pain.

Ed and I knew that the only way to ask intelligent questions of the doctors would be to educate ourselves. We read books and pamphlets, spoke to other breast cancer survivors on the phone, and spent hours researching on the internet. I typed "breast cancer" into one of the search engines on the computer. I was overwhelmed with the number of foundations, support groups and information networks that were available. I started with the three that seemed the most basic, The American Cancer Society (www.cancer.org), Cancer Care, Inc. (www.cancercare.org), and Living Beyond Breast Cancer (www.lbbc.org). I gathered information on financial services, educational services, support groups and other programs in my area.

I literally spent days glued to the computer. I couldn't get enough information on nutrition and treatment options. I kept myself so busy that I didn't even allow myself time to cry. One morning I felt the need to cry, but I thought, "I have people coming to visit in an hour, I better not cry now". Another time the phone had been ringing off the walls and I thought, "I have too many people to talk to, I can't cry now". I actually decided to schedule a time to cry, but I couldn't fit it into my day. That may sound odd, but it was true.

Some of the most touching moments were those spent reading letters and e-mails from family and friends expressing their love for me. I was overwhelmed by their compassion and tenderness. People I didn't even know very well wrote to me offering prayers and words of encouragement. I received cards and letters from friends who I had lost contact with over the years. Others started sharing intimate feelings that we had not shared in more than thirty years of friendship.

I would hesitate to say that having cancer is a gift. But, it was becoming clear to me that many gifts and blessings can come from it. It was touching for me to realize that in spite of cancer, I was very blessed.

"The Tears Finally Come"

I continued to see the surgeon every couple of days while waiting for the results of the tests. Each drive to his office meant more bumps in the road and more caressing of the breast. On the first day he took the drain out. Although this was by no means a pleasant experience, it wasn't as bad as I thought it would be. He told me to take a deep breath, and with one pull he had it out. After the doctor left the examination room, Ed asked me if I wanted to see what the drain looked like. I hesitantly said that I did. He opened the trash bin where the doctor had placed the drain. I don't know what I thought it was going to look like, but the size of it almost knocked me to the floor. It was much larger than I had realized. I was thankful that it was no longer attached to me. One of the most difficult things about having the drain was that it constantly interrupted my sleep. Every time I rolled over, I had been afraid that I would yank it right out of my side. After seeing how long it was, I realized that I had worried for nothing.

I had many visits with the surgeon to have him aspirate the area. He would stick a needle into the armpit, and drain out any accumulated fluid. This was not as painful as I had anticipated. Much of the area was still numb because some of the nerves had been cut during surgery. When he first mentioned that I would need to come back to have the area aspirated, I thought that it was going to be a one-time procedure. I thought that he would put the needle in, drain the fluid out and we would be done. No such luck. I had to go back numerous times. Each time I went, there was less fluid to take out.

At each visit the surgeon would check to see how much flexibility and mobility I had in my arm. He expressed disappointment with my progress on a number of occasions. He told me that I would have to get serious about my exercises if I didn't want to get a frozen shoulder and end up in physical therapy. I told him that I would.

During one visit I had the staples removed from the breast and from the armpit. I had been dreading this moment with all of my heart. First he aspirated the area. Then he removed the staples. I focused my eyes on a spot on the ceiling, and pretended that I was anywhere but in a doctor's office having staples removed from one of the most sensitive parts of my body. Most of it, I have to admit, did not hurt. There were one or two staples that were right in the areola (the ring of tissue that surrounds the nipple). Those did hurt. It made me wonder why anyone in their right mind would purposely elect to have their nipples pierced. My feeling about piercing is that it's painful and unnecessary. God, in his wisdom, has already given us holes wherever he thought we would need them.

That night I finally cried. I sat on the couch with Ed's arms around me, and my arms around a box of tissues. I cried out all of the unfairness, all of the fear, and all of the uncertainty. I cried because I felt vulnerable. Four years earlier, I had undergone brain surgery for

Trigeminal Neuralgia. The year after that, I lost my best friend when she was hit by a car while riding her bicycle. Then came the tragedy of September 11th. Now this.

I was feeling vulnerable and scared. Many of us tend to go through life thinking that we have all the time in the world to achieve our dreams and goals. We go through life thinking that we are healthy and always will be. We go through life thinking we are untouchable.

Cancer changed all that for me.

I cried in Ed's arms until I had no tears left. I felt exhausted physically, emotionally and spiritually. I was tired of hurting. I was tired of talking about this stupid disease. I was tired of people treating me differently than they had just weeks before. I was tired of saying prayers that I wasn't sure anyone was hearing. I was just tired.

"Exit Stage II"

I used to think there could be no more dreaded doctor in the world than the dentist. I was wrong. Looking for an oncologist, the doctor who would treat my cancer, was a surreal experience, to say the least. I was still trying to come to grips with the fact that I had a life-threatening illness. I was not ready for the huge step of calling and making an appointment with a "cancer doctor", yet that's what I needed to do. I wanted to start treatment as quickly as possible to get this disease behind me.

From all of my reading, and from talking to other breast cancer survivors, I knew that I was facing chemotherapy, then radiation, followed by 5 years on a drug called Tamoxifen. Before the visit with the oncologist, I looked at wigs, hats, and bandanas. I knew that going bald was one of the side effects of chemotherapy, so I got myself mentally prepared for it as best I could. I knew in my heart that there was nothing I could do to prepare myself for the moment when I would look in the mirror and see a bald woman with one deformed, scarred breast starring back at me.

A friend of mine had gone through treatments for breast cancer a few years earlier. She highly recommended the oncology group that she had used. She gave me the phone number and I called to make an appointment.

After taking blood and giving me a brief examination, the oncologist brought Ed and me into his office. He sat across the desk from us, and proceeded to give us horrendous news. He said that, although my bone scan and the CT scans of the abdomen and pelvis were clear, my chest CT scan showed that the cancer had spread to both of my lungs.

I don't know how I kept from crying. This nightmare seemed to be getting worse every step of the way. As far as I was concerned, the oncologist had just told me that I was going to die. He said things like: "We'll help you lead as normal a life as possible", and "We'll give you treatments that will allow you to be comfortable for as many years as possible", and "We'll give you the best quality of life that we can."

"SOMEBODY WAKE ME UP!!" This couldn't be real. Ed later told me that he tried his hardest not to look at me for fear that he would break down and cry.

Luckily (yes there is a luckily in all of this) Ed and I had read on the Internet that if the cancer had spread to the lungs, it would NOT mean that I have lung cancer. It would mean that breast cancer cells had moved into the lungs. It would be easier to treat than lung cancer itself.

The oncologist informed us that I had stage IV cancer, not stage II.

Having researched quite extensively, I knew that there were only stages 0-IV. I was at the end of the scale. The wrong end.

The one bright spot in all of this was the oncologist himself. He delivered the news in a calm, professional manner that helped to put me at ease. He allowed Ed and I all the time we needed to process what he was saying and to ask as many questions as needed. He also displayed a very caring and tender side of himself, letting us know that he hated to tell us the news as much as we hated to hear it. I felt a strong connection to this doctor. I felt that I could share a trusting and honest relationship with him. (I wasn't disappointed).

He said that, as the cancer had already spread, I would not have chemotherapy or radiation. I would start taking Tamoxifen right away.

"So let me get this straight," I said. "We are at a more serious stage of this thing, but the treatment is a third of what you would do for stage II?"

He said that is the paradox. For a later stage cancer, the treatment is easier. If it had remained stage II cancer, I would have started chemotherapy and then gone on to radiation and Tamoxifen. Now that "the horse is out of the barn", (the cancer has already spread), the treatment is just Tamoxifen.

I asked him no less than 4 times to explain this rationale. Each time I asked, he calmly explained, never making me feel stupid or uncomfortable. Tamoxifen, he explained, is a type of hormone therapy. It is an estrogen blocker that will starve the cells of estrogen.

"So, no chemo?" I asked again.

"That's right."

"No radiation?"

"No radiation."

"I just take a pill a day?"

"Correct."

That night I cried for the second time. Same couch, same open arms, different box of tissues.

I got the prescription for Tamoxifen filled. I was hoping that it would be a large, nasty-looking pill. I wanted it to look mean and ugly. Instead, it looked like nothing more than an ordinary aspirin. It was small and innocent looking…damn!

Being a snowbird, I would have two oncologists, one in New York and one in Florida.

Most snowbirds carry pictures of their children and grandchildren in their wallets. I carried business cards. I had gynecologist's cards, surgeon's cards, breast specialist's cards, and oncologist's cards. I had business cards for doctors in Florida and doctors in New York. I had cards from hospitals, labs, and private offices. I'd much rather have had pictures of my nieces and nephews.

One of the most painful aspects of dealing with this disease was seeing how my bad news affected other people. I knew it wasn't my fault that I had cancer. I knew that no one saw it as my fault. Yet I couldn't help but feel guilty for the pain I imagined I was causing. I thought about my husband, my parents, my siblings, my nieces, and nephews. I didn't want to bring sadness into their lives, yet there was nothing that I could do to stop it. When I shared these thoughts with Ed, he would remind me that I was not a villain in this. I was a victim. I knew that what he said was true. Still, it was difficult to relate this news to others, hear the pain in their voices, and feel that I was the cause of their pain.

"Pray For Stage II"

Against the better judgment of well-meaning family and friends, we moved back down to Florida for the winter. I heard through the grapevine that some people were asking what I was running away from by going to Florida. They felt that New York had better doctors and better facilities and that it was foolish of me to leave. They didn't understand that I wasn't running away from anything. You don't run away from cancer once it enters your life. Cancer would come with me wherever I went. I didn't have my head in the sand. I knew painfully well that I was dealing with a life-threatening illness. I was extremely grateful for the concern that everyone showed, but my goal at that time was to get to the place where I knew I would heal the best. That place was my own home in sunny Florida.

On December 5th, two days after my 42nd birthday, I met with an oncologist in Florida. My biggest fear was that he would not agree with the course of treatment that the doctor from New York had prescribed. If that were to happen, I would be caught in between two professionals who would be trying to decide the best course of action for, literally, saving my life.

The oncologist examined me and read all of the reports from New York. He told Ed and me that he was not convinced that my cancer was stage IV.

"WHAT??"

"Those spots on the lungs could be anything." He said. "For all we know, it could be scarring from past colds."

He said that he wanted to be absolutely sure that what we were dealing with was stage IV cancer before we continued to treat it as such.

I couldn't believe it. My emotions had been played with so much throughout the past 2 months; I no longer knew what to feel. Many breast cancer survivors had told me that the most difficult part of the ordeal is the time between diagnosis and treatment, when you're not sure what you have and how it will be treated. Unfortunately, I seemed to be stuck in that gray area.

I was confused and upset, but I was also thankful that the oncologist was being thorough. I felt as comfortable with him as I had with the New York oncologist. He had a very pleasant personality and I felt that I could trust him.

The oncologist explained that if the tests showed that it was, in fact, stage II, I would have to stop the hormone therapy, and go on chemotherapy, radiation, and then Tamoxifen. If it were stage IV, I would continue hormone therapy. If the worst-case scenario happened, and we didn't know which it was…well, we'd cross that bridge when, and if, we came to it.

He advised me to go for a PET scan, since that could possibly confirm that it was stage IV. PET stands for Positron Emission Tomography. The doctor explained that a PET scan looks at how much glucose is being used by a tissue. He said that all tissues need glucose to survive. Cancers use more glucose than normal tissues so the scan would light up any "Hot Spots" of activity in my body. I didn't quite understand it then, and I'm not sure that I understand it any better now. I put my trust in the doctor and made an appointment for the following Monday.

First, I was seated in a lounge chair while I was intravenously given a special type of radioactive tracer. Yes, you heard me right, radioactive. I was actually told that I wouldn't be able to be near pregnant women or infants for 2 hours after the test. I felt like I should be glowing. I expected my pee to have an aura to it.

After the injection, I was told to sit quietly for 40 minutes, (which isn't easy for me), while the tracer went through my body. Then I was told to lie on a table as I was put through the PET machine. This meant that I needed to stay absolutely still for another 40 minutes. Of course, as soon as I knew that I wouldn't be able to scratch an itch for almost an hour, I began to feel as if an army of ants was crawling all over my body. It's funny how the mind plays tricks on you.

The PET scan was painless. Not as claustrophobic as an MRI, but not as open as a CT scan.

I was left with the agonizing process of waiting until my next appointment before I would know the results. I told the oncologist that I didn't know what to pray for. Stage II cancer would be less serious than stage IV, but I dreaded the thought of going through months of chemotherapy and radiation, and all of their side effects. Stage IV cancer would certainly be more serious, but the treatments would be easier. The oncologist said, "Pray for stage II."

I did some research on the various stages of cancer so that I would know what I was praying for. It was difficult to grasp everything I read. There was a lot of medical jargon that I wasn't familiar with. Basically,

I learned that the stages have to do with how large the tumor is, if the cancer has spread inside the breast, and if it had spread to nearby tissues, or other organs. I read that stage IV would mean that the cancer had already spread to distant sites such as the bones or lungs, or to lymph nodes not near the breast. I took the doctors advice and prayed for stage II.

We returned to the doctor on December 12th. As soon as he walked through the door of the examination room, I could tell that he did not have good news. He walked over and started to rub my back. Nice gesture. Bad sign.

The PET scan confirmed that the cancer had indeed spread to both of my lungs. Unfortunately, that wasn't the end of the bad news. The scan also showed that the cancer was in the bones in my hips, spine, and chest wall. There was also a spot on my ribs on the left side of my body AND in a lymph node on the left side of my neck. (The same lymph node that in 2000 I asked a doctor to look at. The doctor looked at it and said...you guessed it... "It's nothing to worry about".)

How could this be? My bone scan had been negative for cancer! How could it have spread so much without being detected? Why didn't I have any symptoms? How could this happen to someone who eats all the right foods, exercises regularly, and doesn't smoke? I could be the poster child for the type of person who should not get cancer. Yet the test showed that the cancer had spread far beyond the breast. How long had I been living with this disease without knowing it was there? And, my most pressing question, what were we going to do to get rid of it?

The oncologist said that I should continue with the Tamoxifen to block any estrogen that was lurking about in my system. At the same time, I would start on a medication called Zometa. Being that the cancer had gone to the bones, my skeleton would be susceptible to fractures and breaks. Zometa, which is given by a fifteen-minute intravenous drip once a month, would strengthen the bones.

I asked him when the treatments would begin. He said, "How about right now?"

He instructed one of his nurses to take me to the third floor where I would receive my first treatment of Zometa.

I was taken into the room where the chemotherapy was administered. I was very nervous going into "the chemo room". I felt that I didn't belong there. This room was for sick people. I was young and healthy. What was I doing in a room filled with cancer patients?

I looked around the room and saw at least one dozen chairs lining the walls. Next to each chair was a pole from which anywhere from one to three clear plastic bags were hanging. Some bags had clear liquid in them. Some bags had red liquid in them. Some bags had blue liquid in them. The tubes and needles from these bags were attached to the people in the chairs. I saw needles inserted into arms, the backs of hands and wrists, and into chests. I had read that some people get a port put into their chest. The chemo is then administered through the port, thus putting less wear and tear on the veins.

It was all that I could do to keep from crying. I didn't want to stare at anyone for fear of appearing rude, but I couldn't help myself. I felt as if I were looking into my future. Most of the women in the room were bald. All of the men were bald. Some were sleeping. Some were reading. Some were staring blankly into space. Looking into their eyes, I saw a mixture of emotions. Mostly what I saw was quiet resignation. This had become routine for many of them. They had come to grips with the reality of dealing with cancer, and they went through their treatments without blinking an eye.

I wasn't at that point. This was all new to me, and I was scared. The nurses were pleasant and tried to keep everyone's spirits up. Some of the patients were even laughing and joking around. I wasn't ready for laughter. I just wanted to get the treatment over with. I wanted to leave that room and get on with my life.

After sitting for fifteen minutes, which felt like hours, it was over. I was instructed to return in one month for my next treatment. At that time I would also receive a shot of another medication called Zoladex. The purpose of the Zoladex would be to stop all estrogen production and put me into chemically induced menopause. Zoladex would be administered by a large needle that would insert a pellet into my abdomen. The fun never ends!

"Zometa Hell !!!"

When I was first diagnosed, I read the statistics on the 5-year survival rate for women with breast cancer. For stage II the 5-year survival rate was 80%. For stage IV it was 22%. My odds had gone down drastically.

It was time to make more phone calls and spread more bad news. I tried to keep my voice as upbeat and cheerful as possible. How do you prepare yourself to tell your mother and father that their daughter has a 22% chance of being alive in five years? How do you prepare yourself to tell people that cancer, perhaps the most dreaded disease in the world, has further invaded your body? I found that there was no way to prepare. You just pick up the phone, take a deep breath and do it.

I called my parents first. They handled the news better than I could have hoped. Their main concern was for Ed and me and our reaction to all that had happened. I wasn't sure if they were being strong for my benefit, or if I was being strong for theirs. Probably a little of both.

Immediately upon hearing my news they offered to come to my house with dinner. My Mother and Father were fellow snowbirds. They lived in Port St. Lucie, only thirty minutes from Jensen Beach. I appreciated their offer and teased them about being my own personal meals on wheels. When they came over that night, Ed and I filled them in on everything the oncologist said. I felt very protective of their feelings and tried my hardest to keep the conversation as light as possible. I tried to point out as many hopeful and optimistic aspects of the situation as I could, but there weren't many. My parents made me promise that I would be honest with them and not hide anything from them. I promised. They were a terrific source of strength and support and I felt comforted to have them by my side.

After my parents left, I called my brother and my sisters. After filling them in on the news and answering any questions they had, I said, "OK, now let's talk about anything but cancer." Loretta told me about the repairs that she and her husband, Jimmy, were making to their house. My brother George, and his wife Mary, filled me in on their jobs and told me some new jokes. Grace and her husband, Paul, talked to me about their children and their dogs.

I spoke with my eight nieces and nephews. The girls, Katie, Allison, Kara, Valerie, and Teresa talked with me about proms, school, and sweet sixteen parties. The boys, Anthony, Christopher, and Jamie talked with me about karate, soccer and baseball. It felt so good to hear their stories and laugh with them. Cancer dominated my life ever since I was diagnosed. How good it felt to take a break from that and laugh again.

Ed and I also spoke with Amy, her husband Ricky, Marcia, and her husband Bernie. They all sent their love, positive thoughts and prayers. They expressed frustration at being so far away from us. They all wanted to help, but didn't know how from such a distance. I told them that they were helping just by being on the other end of the phone. Staying connected to family and friends was so important to me at that time. I was lucky to have so much family that I also considered friends.

Unfortunately, the laughter and good feelings didn't last for long. That night all hell broke loose. I woke up in the middle of the night with a temperature that kept soaring and dropping and soaring back up again. Every bone in my body ached like never before. I couldn't stop sweating. I had chills. My teeth were chattering. All that I was able to do was lie in one position and moan. I don't know why, but moaning felt comforting to me. Ed rubbed my back, got aspirin for me and put compresses on my head. At one point during the night I looked at him and asked, "Is this it?" I had heard stories about people dying within weeks of being diagnosed with cancer. I thought I might be one of those people. Ed told me that I was just feeling the effects of the new medication. Days later he told me that he was just as afraid as I was. He told me that he spent the whole night lying awake feeling my breath on his cheek, praying that the breaths would keep coming.

The following morning I called the doctor. He said that what I experienced was normal for people just starting Zometa. He instructed me to take Tylenol for the fever and for the pain. I made him promise that I wasn't going to experience this every month. He promised. (I'm happy to report that the doctor was true to his word. I never experienced a reaction like that again.)

I had been having headaches for quite some time. The doctor said that I should have an MRI of the brain to see if the cancer had gone there. An appointment was set for the following Monday. More testing. More waiting.

Ed and I took all of this news like troopers. We went out to lunch. We went Christmas shopping. We bought ourselves some CD's. Then we went home and cried.

I had had many MRI's of my brain while I was being tested and treated for Trigeminal Neuralgia. I felt certain that if there had been cancer in my brain, one of those tests would have picked it up. However, in the past months I had 2 mammograms fail to pick up a large tumor in my breast, and I had a bone scan fail to detect at least half a dozen cancerous tumors in my bones. Even though I like and trust all of my doctors, I was rapidly losing faith in the medical profession's testing procedures.

On December 19th, Ed and I met with the oncologist and received our first piece of good news in over 2 months. The MRI of the brain showed no signs of cancer. I wanted to rejoice. I wanted to trust this morsel of good news that we had been given. Yet, in my heart, I felt that the results were not written in stone. I knew that I needed to have faith. I had enough on my plate as it was. I didn't need the stress of second-guessing each and every test. Besides, whether the cancer had gone to the brain or not, the course of treatment would remain the same.

Ed and I made more phone calls. This time we were able to give everyone good news.

We spent that Christmas in Florida. We wanted to be in New York with our families, but I was unable to fly. I had been told that there was a 50-50 chance that the change in cabin pressure on the plane would cause lymphedema. I couldn't take the chance. Also, I was concerned about all of the germs on the plane. My resistance was low. I would be risking infection by being around so many people in a confined area, especially during cold and flu season. Cancer had taken another important part of my life away from me.

From December 2002 until March 2003 my treatments were pretty simple. I took Tamoxifen once a day. Once a month I received my IV of Zometa and my injection of Zoladex.

I stopped getting my period in February 2003, which meant that I was losing estrogen and starving those nasty little cancer cells. It also meant that I was in menopause. Aside from the hot flashes, which I started to refer to as power surges, the side effects were minimal. That isn't to minimize hot flashes. I used to think that women exaggerated the intensity of these flashes. I was wrong. It didn't feel like I was getting hot from the outside. The heat was coming from inside of me… and it was intense. The flashes were preceded by a "panicky" feeling. This was particularly disturbing at night when I was trying to sleep. I would start to drift off to dreamland, and then suddenly I would feel jumpy. My pulse would start to race and I felt like I was sinking into a black hole of depression. Seconds later it would feel as if I was burning from the inside out. Off went the blanket. Off went the sheets. Off went Ed's arm from around my waist. Off went the pajamas. I couldn't cool down fast enough. Within no time at all I would feel cold. On went the pajamas. On went Ed's arm. On went the sheets. On went the blanket. This would happen numerous times throughout the night making it impossible to sleep.

Although I was losing sleep, wearing out the threads on my sheets and ripping Ed's shoulder out of it's socket every night, there was good news. My symptoms were improving. My hip, which had caused me to walk with a limp, stopped hurting, and I was back to walking normally again. The lymph node on the side of my neck had decreased greatly in size. My cough, which seemed to have come out of nowhere, was gone. I was swimming again, going for long walks and feeling energetic for the first time in months.

I saw the oncologist once a month for a physical examination and he seemed to be happy with my progress. I was optimistic that I had this dreaded disease under control.

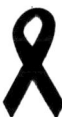

"More Tests...More Waiting"

I had my next doctor's appointment on the first day of spring. I had been experiencing some pain on the left side of my lower back. I attributed it to the fact that I was overly ambitious one day, cleaning out closets and lifting heavy boxes. I wasn't worried about it being due to the cancer.

The oncologist, however, wasted no time giving us some serious news. My tumor marker was once again elevated. He said that he didn't want to alarm us because these markers can fluctuate. It only becomes a problem if there is an upward trend over time. He said that he wanted more blood drawn so he could see what the markers were reading. He gave me instructions to call him on Tuesday for the results.

I didn't feel good about this. I wanted to keep my optimism going, but I just didn't feel right. The pain in my back was getting worse, and I was feeling more tired than usual. Ed and I tried not to put too much thought into it. Tuesday would be here soon enough. We would deal with whatever news the doctor gave us at that time.

Once again, we had the agonizing experience of waiting. We had grown to understand that although the tests were difficult to endure, and the bad news difficult to take, the truly hard part of this experience was the waiting. It was a helpless feeling. There was no way to push the clock forward. We could not press fast forward like we could on a VCR or DVD player. We just had to occupy ourselves as best we could while waiting for the days to pass.

I called the oncologist. The news was not good. My tumor marker was elevated. The normal range for this particular marker (CA 15-3) is 0-31. (In New York the marker used is the CA 27-29 and the range is 0-38). On December 5th, my marker was 44. Two months later it was 131. The blood test that he took on that first day of Spring showed that my marker had risen to 242. The tests were showing the upward trend that I so badly did not want to see. I knew this meant that I was not responding to treatment and that the cancer was progressing.

I wasted no time asking the oncologist what we needed to do. He said that he would schedule new CT scans and bone scans for me within the next few days. The results of the tests would determine the course of action. He said that if the tests showed changes in the bones, we would try another hormone treatment. If the cancer was affecting internal organs, I would go on chemotherapy.

I knew that thousands of brave men, women and children had endured chemo, but I dreaded the thought of putting those poisons into my body. I have always been a firm believer in exercise and proper nutrition. The thought of putting poisonous chemicals into my body made me nauseous. The thought of going bald upset me. We were planning to start our journey back to New York in only one month. Our plan was to stay with my brother and his family while Ed worked on the boat, getting her ready for another season. Our plans were put on hold as we did what we had grown to hate. We waited.

The doctor scheduled my tests for that Friday. I was not thrilled with the prospect of taking tests whose results I had little faith in, but that was the standard of care. I had little choice. I was scheduled to see the doctor on the following Monday, at which time he would give me the results of the tests and discuss my treatment options with me.

My mother and father joined Ed and me for the next appointment with the oncologist. He explained that I should start chemotherapy because of the rate the cancer had been growing. He told us that my internal organs were OK. However, due to the fact that I responded so poorly to Tamoxifen, he felt that chemo would be my best option to stop the spread of the disease. I asked him what type of chemo I would be going on and what the side effects would be. He explained that the chemo was called Taxotere. The side effects included total hair loss, (within twenty days of beginning treatment), bone pain, and fatigue. Along with Taxotere I would continue on Zometa and Zoladex. The oncologist told me that I would be taking steroids the day before chemo, the day of chemo and the day after. The steroids, he told me, would help my body manage the effects of the drugs.

Being a nut for the Internet, I looked up Taxotere when I got home. I learned that side effects could also include swelling and fluid retention, problems with fingernails and toenails becoming discolored or even falling off, mouth sores, runny or dry eyes, diarrhea or constipation, fuzzy thinking (also known as chemo-brain), a suppressed immune system, and a loss of feeling in hands and feet. (Are we having fun yet???)

I braced myself for my first chemo treatment, which would be on April 3rd.

Once again my parents, Ed and I found ourselves with the dreaded task of making phone calls and writing e-mails to family and friends asking for their prayers, positive thoughts and good energy. I believed that my life had become a soap opera for some people, asking over and over again to PLEASE keep them informed, so we did. Within 24 hours I had 22 e-mails to respond to and a dozen phone calls. I'm not sure that anyone can understand how important words of encouragement are to someone in my situation. Some people started to send me jokes, as they knew of my belief in laughter being the best medicine. Some friends offered prayer services in my name. Others lit candles at their church. Some sent cards and gifts. All of them expressed love and support and outrage that this disease had entered our lives.

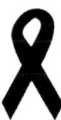

"Chemotherapy Begins"

Knowing that I was going to lose my hair was probably more traumatic for me than any of the other side effects that I read about. I couldn't believe how vain I was being. There I was, facing a deadly disease and my worst fear was going bald.

Ed and I went wig shopping. We walked into only one wig store; tried on only one wig and were amazed at how much it looked like my own hair. We paid $100.00 dollars for the wig. I also learned that the American Cancer Society supplied free wigs for those going through chemo treatments. I didn't use this service, but it was good information to have.

I stocked up on baseball caps, bandanas, hats, and other assorted head coverings. I read a lot of information about "surviving" chemotherapy by getting plenty of rest, eating right, staying well hydrated and exercising as often as your body would allow. I shopped for all of the "healthy" foods such as green, leafy vegetables, plenty of fruit and gallons of water. One woman who had survived stage IV ovarian cancer told me to start drinking wheat grass juice. Another told me to buy a good juicer. I was ready to try anything that I thought might work. I stocked up on wheat grass and bought myself the best juicer money could buy.

I packed a bag of goodies to take to the chemo session with me. I had books, relaxing music, a bottle of water, mints, a sleeve of crackers and pen and paper just in case I got inspired to write. It looked like I was planning to be away for the weekend instead of just a few hours.

I walked into the treatment room on April 3rd feeling absolutely fine and willingly allowed people to hook me up to poisonous substances, knowing that they would make me feel like hell for the next week. (What's wrong with this picture?)

A line of chairs was placed against a wall across from a set of windows overlooking the Intracoastal Waterway; the same Intracoastal Waterway that only five years ago Ed and I had been sailing on without a care in the world. How I wished I were back on our boat instead of sitting where I was, dealing with what I was dealing with.

The nurse "hooked me up" to my bags of medications. She put a large needle into one of the veins in the back of my hand. This wasn't easy considering the fact that I have very small veins. She had to try 3 times before getting it to hold. The nurse informed me that the woman sitting next to me was on the same chemotherapy as me. I asked the woman about the side effects. She told me about the loss of hair including eyebrows, eyelashes, and pubic hair. She also said that for a few days after therapy I would feel as though I had been run over by a truck. Now, there's something to look forward to.

I set my book, my pen and paper, my headphones and my water bottle on the small table next to my chair. I didn't use any of them. Along with the chemo, I was given Benadryl to help lessen the effects of the chemo. The Benadryl put me right to sleep. I guess that's a good thing. If you have to go through a miserable experience, why not sleep your way through it?

I woke up feeling weak and woozy. Ed drove me home and I waited for the effects of the chemo to hit.

That first day wasn't so bad. The second day wasn't too bad either. My face was flushed and felt hot. I knew that was due to the steroids. I had more energy than I expected to have. No nausea, no bone pain, no fatigue. I thought that this chemo thing wouldn't be so bad after all.

"Oh...My...God!!!"

When the woman in the chemo room told me that I would feel as though I had been run over by a truck, she failed to tell me just how big that truck would be, and how fast it would be going. I woke up the following morning to feel pain in muscles and joints I didn't even know I had. My neck was sore. I could barely lift my legs high enough to go up the stairs. My arms felt heavy and stiff. My face was red and puffy, and my eyes felt as if they were being cut by shards of glass. (Other than that, it was a good day.)

Fortunately, or unfortunately, the oncologist said that these were all normal reactions to the chemotherapy. I didn't feel nauseous and for that I was thankful. I couldn't imagine the pain my body would be in if I were convulsing with nausea on top of everything else.

A few days later I woke to a new surprise. Parts of my neck and back were filled with itchy, stinging, red pimples. I called the oncologist. He told me to come in right away. After examining me, he said that it looked like I had a case of shingles. I could have cried. I was so

136

frustrated. My bones hurt. My skin was itchy. I was tired, but couldn't sleep. I wasn't able to eat the kinds of foods that I knew I should be eating. I didn't want fruit. I wanted lasagna. I didn't want vegetables. I wanted macaroni and cheese. I didn't want to drink the gallon of water that I knew I needed to drink to help pass the chemicals through my system. Now I had shingles. How in the world was I going to go through this every time I had chemotherapy?

The doctor assured me that this was an unusual reaction. He said that he wanted to have blood drawn to see how high, or low, my white blood count was. After having the blood drawn and tested, the oncologist said that my white blood count was "dangerously" low, leaving me at risk of further infection. He said that he could give me an injection to bring the white blood count up, but he had two concerns. The first concern was whether or not my insurance would cover the injection, which costs thousands of dollars. The second concern was that the medication, called Neulasta, would cause a lot of bone pain. I didn't think that I could stand any more bone pain, but I understood that it would be a huge risk to allow the blood count to remain so low.

My insurance company did cover the shot. I got the shot.

The following day I was miserable with bone pain on top of bone pain. I had read that the effects of chemotherapy do not get easier over time. In fact, I read that the effects become cumulative, and I was in it for the long haul. I prayed that what I read was not true for everyone. I prayed long and hard that I was experiencing the worst of it and that it would only get easier.

Twenty days later, as promised, my hair started to fall out. My scalp hurt, which I wasn't expecting. I didn't know that there would be pain involved in my hair loss, but there was. I had gotten a super short hair cut just days before my twenty-day deadline was up. I had heard that it would be traumatic to see my hair fall out. The shorter the hair, the easier it would be emotionally. The first thing to go was my pubic hair. I was in the shower one morning. As soon as the spray of water hit that area, the hair just fell off and headed for the drain. I found myself following it yelling, "Where ya going?? Come back here!!" Looking back, I have to laugh, although at the time it was more pathetic than funny.

I found myself mesmerized by the process of balding. One night I watched TV with a paper plate on my lap. I ran my fingers through my hair and watched it rain onto the plate. I also let my hair fall into the sink in various designs and patterns. I tried to amuse myself with this tragic event, but it wasn't very amusing. I got tired of finding hair on pillowcases, in shower drains, on the kitchen floor, and all over my clothes. I asked Ed to shave my head for me.

I thought that I was emotionally prepared to see myself bald…I wasn't. Without hair on top of my head, on my eyebrows or on my eyelashes, I looked like an alien from outer space. Ed and I did our best to keep our sense of humor. We joked about coloring my head for Easter or painting eyes on the back of my head. We did a good job of staying upbeat most of the time, but my baldness had a serious affect on how I saw myself. Let's face it, it's hard to feel sexy or feminine when you look like Mr. Clean in drag. By the way, did I mention that the fuzzy hairs on my chin and upper lip stayed put? **WHAT…IS…UP… WITH…THAT??**

My parents came over that night. I wanted them to be the first ones to see my hairless head. I was embarrassed to show them, but not as badly as I thought I would be. I was happy to see that neither of them looked shocked. Their calm reaction helped me know that even though I saw myself differently, they didn't. We ate dinner, laughed, and talked as if nothing had changed.

In time I was able to take my wig off in front of some of my friends without feeling like a freak. I knew that there was nothing "freaky" about being bald because of chemotherapy. I just couldn't shake the feeling that I was wearing a neon sign on top of my head that said, "Hey, look at me! I have cancer!" Before going bald, no one would have noticed that there was anything wrong with me. I looked toned, tan and healthy. Now I felt that it was the first and only thing people noticed about me.

My first three rounds of chemotherapy were filled with side effects that I had been warned about, but still was not prepared for. My eyes felt like they were filled with sand most of the time. I used artificial tears to combat this, but it only helped a little. I developed a rash with each round of chemo and stayed up nights laying in a warm oatmeal bath. My nails turned yellow and brown and separated from the nail beds. This was not only unsightly. It was horribly painful. I was afraid of losing the nails altogether, but luckily I never did. I experienced bone pain, sleeplessness, weight gain, dry skin, and oral thrush. The oncology nurses, as well as other cancer patients, were able to give me remedies to combat all of the side effects that I experienced.

I spent a lot of time those first few weeks crying and praying. Sometimes I would want to have Ed by my side as I cried. More often, I wanted to be alone to cry out my fear, my frustration and my anger. I wanted to be alone to feel sorry for myself, to curse, scream, beg and ask, "Why me?" I wanted to be alone to face the possibility of imminent death for the first time in my life.

We all know that we're going to die. Suddenly I was forced to come face to face with the possibility that death may come sooner than I ever could have imagined. I started to wonder what it would actually be like to be in Heaven. Is there a Heaven? Would I meet God? Would he be proud of the way I had lived my life? Would he approve of the way that I handled my illness and my death? What would my funeral be like? Do I want to have a funeral? Who would come to say their final good-bye? These thoughts invaded my every waking hour and interrupted my much-needed sleep.

My biggest concern was leaving Ed. I couldn't imagine living my life without him. It was painful to think about him living his life without me. I cried for him, as much as, if not more than, for myself. I cried for my parents, my siblings, my nieces and nephews and all of my family and friends. I cried because I didn't want to die, but I didn't want to live with the pain of cancer either.

I spent a great deal of time putting on my "happy face" when I was with other people. I wanted so badly to be the old me, the fun me, the carefree me. I wanted to act as if nothing had changed, when in reality everything had. My family expressed concern over my lack of sadness and anger towards this disease. I assured them that I was sad and I was angry. I just chose to attend to those feelings in private.

I became extremely aware of my body. Every new ache or pain made me think that the cancer was growing. I thought every pimple was cancer. Anytime that I developed a cough, I was sure it was cancer. I felt a little foolish running to the doctor with every symptom that appeared, but I didn't care. I would rather appear foolish than miss mentioning something that might be important.

I kept a daily journal detailing the severity and location of my pains. I also rated my days on a scale of 1-10.

1- I feel great today. Plenty of energy. No pain at all.

2- I feel good. I have some energy. Not much pain.

3- I've been better, but I really can't complain.

4- I have a little pain, but nothing terrible. Wish I had more energy.

5- I'm a little sluggish today. Pains are coming and going.

6- I have just enough energy to get frustrated by all the things I can't do.

7- I'm not feeling so good. Pretty tired throughout the day. More pain than usual.

8- I have a lot of pain today. Zero energy. I don't feel good at all.

9- Holy crap!

10- Is suicide legal in this state?

I also kept a notebook of questions that I wanted to ask the doctor during my next visit. Questions like:

-What are the names of the drugs that I'm taking?

-What are the side effects?

-Should I avoid certain foods, beverages or activities?

-Will it affect my sex life?

-How will this treatment affect my internal organs?

-Will I experience weight gain, hair loss, fatigue, vomiting?

-How can I reduce my risk of side effects?

The list grew every day. The more I read, the more questions I had. The doctors and nurses never hesitated to answer all of my questions, listen to all of my concerns and encourage me to keep asking as many questions as I needed to. I was grateful for their patience and sensitivity. These doctors and nurses who help people cope with cancer every day are true angels in my book.

"Support Group"

In the course of my research I learned that, statistically, people who attended support groups had a better survival rate than those who did not attend support groups. I wasn't sure why this was true. However, I was ready to do anything that I thought might increase my chances of survival. If someone told me that kissing pigs would increase my chances of surviving cancer, I would have stocked up on lip balm, puckered up, and sat in the middle of the largest pig farm I could find.

With this in mind, I set out to find a group in my area. Most of the groups that I found were for people much older than me. Some of the groups were not limited to breast cancer. They were for men and women with all kinds of cancers. I wasn't interested in listening to people's battles with prostate cancer, lung cancer or brain cancer. I was glad to see that there were groups available for people with these forms of cancer, but my needs were very specific. I wanted to find a group for women in their 40's with stage IV breast cancer. I wanted to find a group of people who would be able to relate to what I was going through.

Stage IV turned out to be a lonely place. I could not find a single group for people with stage IV cancer. One day I saw a flyer in the doctor's office for a group called "For the young and the young at heart". The name caught my attention. I called the American Cancer Society and they gave me information on where and when the group met.

As a Social Worker I had facilitated many groups: groups for children of divorced parents, groups for teenaged parents, groups for boys, groups for girls and groups for adults. I had run many support groups, but I had never been a participant. This would be my first time experiencing the anxiety, excitement, nervousness, and fear that come with attending a support group. I was going to be the new kid on the block. I knew that I would be expected to share feelings that were personal and private to me. I wasn't sure I was ready to do that.

I wasn't even sure if a group would be right for me. Did I really want to listen to other people's experiences with this awful disease? Did I really want to relive the shock of being diagnosed and the pain of the surgeries? Did I want to talk month after month about life-threatening topics? I decided to attend the first meeting. If I didn't like it, I would be under no obligation to go back again.

Twelve women, ranging in age from early 20's to 60's sat around a long table in one of the conference rooms of a local hospital. Some participants were newly diagnosed, while some had been cancer free for as much as 4 years. Some women had lumpectomies. Some women had mastectomies. Some of the women were diagnosed with stage I cancer and one...God bless her...one woman was diagnosed with stage IV. I was no longer alone. At least one other person knew how I felt. A few of the women had negative side effects from chemotherapy. They openly shared what worked best for them in managing these effects. One woman said that her eyes would not stop watering. Another member of the group had experienced the same thing. She said that her eyes were watery, believe it or not, because they were dry. The chemo was causing her eyes to dry out so her tear ducts were working overtime to help them stay moist. She said that she used an over-the-counter artificial tear solution and it worked for her.

Another woman, whose hair was thinning because of chemotherapy, said that she was tired of finding hair on her pillowcase every morning. She was told to try a silk or satin pillowcase instead of cotton. The silk and satin materials are smoother on the scalp, thus causing less friction on the hair. (I tried this myself. Satin pillowcases really helped to lessen the amount of hair that came out during the night.)

I asked if anyone had experienced itchy, red rashes on their buttocks as a side effect. No one had. We had quite a laugh as I described my visit to the doctor to show him my rash.

I went into the examination room and told the doctor my symptoms; a red rash on my buttocks and anus. He said that he needed to see the rash.

"Why do you need to see it?"

"So I know how to treat it."

"It's a red rash. Give me a pencil and a red crayon, I'll draw it for you."

"I need to see what kind of rash it is or I won't know what to prescribe for you."

"So, I need to drop my pants so you can look at my butt?"

"Yes. And your anus."

"You're kidding!"

"No, I'm not."

"IT'S THE SAME RASH!!"

"Are you going to cooperate? I have other patients to see."

"OK. I'll do it, but who...you know...who...spreads the cheeks?"

"Would you prefer that I do it?"

"Hell, no!!"

"Then you'll have to."

I oh-so-slowly unbuttoned my pants, lowered them to my knees and bent over the examination table.

"Um, Laura?"

"Yes, doctor."

"I can't see through your underpants. They'll have to come down too."

I oh-so-slowly lowered my underpants. I believe that my face turned redder than my butt. The doctor looked at the rash on my buttocks.

"OK, now the anus."

I reached around either side of my buttocks and grabbed hold of each cheek.

"I can't do it."

"Then move your hands, I'll do it."

"No, wait. I'll do it myself."

I reached around and grabbed hold of each cheek again.

"I just can't do it!!" I was laughing at this point. What else could I do?

By this time the doctor had lost his patience. He gently parted the seas, took a quick look and within less than a second it was over. He prescribed a cream for me and told me to continue with the warm oatmeal baths.

The women laughed hysterically at my story. They laughed even harder when they told me who the guest speaker at our next meeting was going to be. None other than my butt doctor. It felt good to find humor in an otherwise embarrassing situation.

For two hours we asked each other questions, we shared our feelings, and we traded "survival techniques" as if they were recipes. We talked about sexuality, pain management, and sleep disorders.

We laughed together. We encouraged each other. I found the group to be a refreshing and comfortable place to share my thoughts and have my questions answered. I felt safe. I learned why people who attend support groups have an increased survival rate. For starters, the exchange of information is invaluable. The camaraderie and laughter is refreshing. It is inspiring to hear stories of people who are living full and active lives with cancer. (One woman in the group told us about a friend who had been living with stage IV cancer for eleven years.) Now that's inspiring!

That same winter I met with the editor of a newsletter called TAKING THE FEAR OUT OF CANCER. I told her that I enjoyed reading her newsletter and that I would be interested in submitting an article or two. After reading some of my work she offered me my own column. I happily accepted. The column was titled BREAST CANCER: LIVING BEYOND THE FEAR.

Writing this column was therapy for me. It gave me an incredible sense of power to take this horrible experience and turn it into something positive. I wrote about good nutrition, exercise, and the importance of keeping a good attitude. I wrote about my experience with the support group (leaving out the buttocks/anus story) and encouraged others to seek out a group in their area. I used my Social Work background to help people understand the stages of grieving from denial to acceptance. I wrote about the important role of the caregivers and their need for support. (I believe that the caregivers are the unsung heroes in the fight against cancer.)

I had an article titled, "Talk To Your Cancer", published in COPING magazine. As a Social Worker I used to encourage clients to write letters to the people and things in their lives that caused them pain. They wrote letters to alcoholic parents, abusive spouses, and to their addictions. This was an activity that was solely for the benefit of the client. It was a way for them to release their pent-up feelings in a totally safe environment. The letters were never actually sent. In fact, they were usually destroyed right after being written. This allowed the client freedom to be as honest as they wanted to be, secure in knowing that no one would ever see what they had written. In the article I encouraged people living with cancer to write letters and poems to their diseases. I encouraged them to be as honest with their feelings as they could be. I believe this exercise provides a wonderful sense of power over people and things that we might otherwise feel powerless over. It is a form of cleansing. A catharsis.

After having the article published I decided to take my own advice. I started to write letters to my cancer. In my writings I expressed feelings of anger, fear, and rage along with feelings of strength and determination. Those writings would become the inspiration for DEAR CANCER.

"Back To New York"

In May, Ed and I traveled back to New York. I presented my hairless head to the rest of my family and to my friends for the first time. I was terribly afraid of what the children would say. I was afraid that they would be embarrassed to be seen with me. I was afraid that they would forget, "fun Aunt Laura", and just see me as a sickly person to avoid and fear. I was angry at the timing of my baldness. I had spent much of my winter in Florida feeling good. Why was it now, when I was returning home for a summer of backyard barbeques and boating, that I had to be going through so many rounds of chemotherapy? Then again, is there ever a good time to go through chemotherapy?

My fears of the children's reactions proved to be silly. They handled it beautifully. I arrived at Grace's house in New Jersey to be greeted by her and her daughter Kara, wearing plastic, flesh-colored coverings on their heads making them look bald. I arrived at my brother's house to see him, his wife and three children wearing wigs that they had bought just for my arrival. It made me laugh. Mostly, it made me happy to see that they knew "fun Aunt Laura" would have maintained her sense of humor. I found that as long as I was at ease with my baldness, they were at ease with it. I wore the wig the majority of the time. I revealed my bald head to them when I thought that they, and I, were ready for it. They thought it was funny and even got a kick out of rubbing my head for luck.

I found the wig to be incredibly itchy and hot during the summer months and opted to wear either a bandana or a baseball cap. I protected my skin by wearing a large hat, a long-sleeve cover-up and plenty of suntan lotion. At the beach, my friends made sure that I had a shady spot under a large umbrella at all times. I took naps when I needed them. I timed my chemotherapy treatments so that they wouldn't interfere with any parties or family gatherings. (I lost a lot to cancer, but I didn't lose my priorities.) I tried to keep my life as normal as possible. I was fortunate to have a husband, family and friends to help me maintain that.

I continued treatments with the New York oncologist. During one visit I asked him how long I would have to remain on chemotherapy. He explained that as my cancer was stage IV, I would probably be on it for the rest of my life. He said I would be able to take chemo holidays, (or chemo vacations). These would be breaks in my treatment when he would put me on hormone therapy while my body rested from all of the poisons it had endured. If that was going to be my reality, I thought it best to look into having a port put in. As I said earlier, I have small veins and the nurses always have a hard time getting the IV needle into place. It's frustrating and painful.

On May 28, I met with a surgeon who said that he would be able to put in a port-a-cath. He explained that it is a device that is placed under the skin in the chest or arm. Mine would be in the chest. The port is made up of a small metal chamber and a catheter. The tip of the catheter is inserted into a vein just above the heart. During treatments, a specially designed needle is inserted into the port. The medication or fluid flows through the needle, into the port, and through the catheter, directly into the bloodstream.

I had the surgery on June 11. To my surprise, (and delight), I went through the surgery with no problems. I didn't even throw up in the recovery room. The port left a round lump on the left side of my chest just below the collarbone. It was just another constant reminder of the hell that had entered my life.

The port was not too painful, however I did have a problem when I drove my car. The part of the seatbelt that goes over the shoulder sat right on the port, pushing it into my skin. I learned that I could relieve the pressure by placing a small pillow between my body and the seatbelt. The pain only lasted for about one week. After that I was able to wear the seatbelt with no problems.

I was due for my next chemo treatment only two days after the surgery. I was nervous about getting a needle put into the newly "installed" port. The incision was still raw and the area around the port was still sensitive.

I had my treatment and was very happy to find that the needle didn't hurt at all. As a matter of fact, I was waiting for the nurse to put it in when I realized that she already had. The port was unsightly, and looked painful, but it made my treatments a little bit easier. I no longer dreaded the IV needle every 3 weeks. My blood was drawn through the port and all of my treatments were administered through it.

I remained on chemotherapy from April 2003 until August 2004. I was happy to learn that, in my case, the chemo did not have a cumulative effect. In fact, the longer I was on chemotherapy, the better I became at handling the side effects. In the beginning I had my treatments once every 3 weeks. Eventually the time between treatments was increased, and I was going once a month. I could usually count on at least 5 days of lying on the couch with zero energy, but plenty of bone and nerve pain. Many people say that getting chemo once a month feels like getting the flu once a month. I guess that's true, except with chemo there were a lot more side effects.

I tried to remain focused on, and thankful for, the good things. I didn't have much nausea. I was incredibly grateful for that. I had a husband who took excellent care of me. My parents lived close by, and helped get us through some very tough times. My family and Ed's family gave us a great deal of emotional support. I received many cards, e-mails, and phone calls from family and friends. I was still able to go sailing, and take long walks in nature. I went canoeing. I went out dancing with my friends. I even went on my first hot air balloon ride, and saw my favorite performer, Jimmy Buffett, in concert.

My niece Kara had asked me to be her confirmation sponsor. I was honored that she chose me. I wanted her confirmation celebration to be something that she would remember forever. I made plans to have her sleep aboard FREEDOM II, attend the Hampton Classic, (a popular horse show in the Hamptons on Long Island), and go to dinner at one of our favorite restaurants. I was just as excited about the day as Kara. However, in the back of my mind I was afraid that I would not feel well. I was afraid of having my health spoil the celebration for her. (With chemotherapy, I never knew how I would feel from one day to the next.)

Much to my delight, the day turned out fine. I didn't have as much energy as I would have hoped, but Kara had enough for both of us. The following day Kara's parents had a party for her in their backyard in New Jersey. They rented a tent and a dance floor, and hired a DJ for the evening. I wasn't about to let the fact that I was bald and on chemotherapy stop me from dancing. I danced for hours. I knew that my bones would hurt the following day, but I pushed that thought aside and kept right on dancing. If having cancer taught me anything, it was to enjoy every second of every moment of every day. That's just what I planned to do. I made the most of the good times and dealt with the bad times.

I believe that keeping my mind focused on positive people and things helped me through the worst times. So much so, that I made it a point to notice at least 3 positive things every day. Some days it was hard to find 3 things to be grateful for, but I found that if I looked hard enough, I would always find something. Some days my list included such simple things as seeing a butterfly, being able to sit at the table without pain, or sleeping through the night.

On the days when I felt good, I would write articles for my column, work on my book, and get together with friends. I did as much exercise as I could in order to stay in shape. I tried to have as much fun as possible. I didn't want to miss out on one single party because I always had the fear that it could be my last. There were some rare times when I would be sitting with friends, laughing, and for that one moment I would not be thinking about cancer. Those times were precious and few.

It was August 2004 when my oncologist said that I was ready for a chemo holiday. It was time to try hormone therapy. I remembered when I first learned that I would have to go on chemotherapy. I remembered reading that most people have 8 rounds of chemo followed by radiation. 8 rounds sounded like forever to me. I lost count over the months, but I believe I ended up receiving more than 23 chemo treatments. I never had any radiation.

I was more than thrilled to be getting off of the chemo...MUCH more. It was the best news I had gotten in a very long time. I felt as if I had just been given a new lease on life. I was already looking forward to my hair growing back, my energy increasing, and my "chemo brain" going away. I was looking forward to feeling like my old self again.

The new drug was called Femara. I was told that most people were "chemo-free" anywhere from four months to two years on Femara. I prayed that I would get at least a couple of years from it.

The Femara worked well and had very few side effects. The treatment consisted of taking one pill a day. It kept my numbers in the normal range and before long I was starting to feel some of my strength come back. I started to lose the puffiness that I had gotten from the steroids. I watched my weight shrink. I watched my hair grow. It grew back v-e-r-y slowly. At first I had peach fuzz on top of my head. When it started to grow back at a faster pace, I was surprised at the color and the texture. My hair had always been straight. The color was always light brown, (with blonde streaks thanks to artificial hair coloring). What I found growing on my head was curls upon curls of dark, black hair with kinky, gray hairs making me look older than my 44 years.

I continued on Femara. I went to the doctor's office once a month for a check up, to have blood drawn, and to receive an infusion of Zometa. I was taken off of Zoladex and put on a medication called Lupron to keep me in menopause. Lupron was administered by an injection in the hindquarters once a month.

It felt strange coming off of the chemo. I was starting to feel like myself again, yet I wasn't sure who I was anymore. I looked different. I felt different. My sense of humor, which used to be sharp and quick, didn't feel quick anymore. I felt like my mind was always on a slower gear than everyone around me. I tried to explain that it was something called, "chemo brain", but I think most people assumed I was joking. **"Chemo brain" is real**. Research is showing that the chemical activity affecting the brain during chemotherapy causes changes in the way in which the brain functions. Some people don't believe in "chemo brain".

Having been there, I can attest to the fact that it is a real and difficult problem.

I was still taking other medications that caused drowsiness, so I truly wasn't myself. I had been on so many medications for so long that I actually couldn't remember what it felt like to be clear-headed and alert. I had a constant feeling of drowsiness, which I tried to hide most of the time. I was desperate to get back to my "old self".

I had read that the effects of chemotherapy, including the foggy thinking and fuzzy feeling in your head, linger for the same amount of time that you were on chemo. I was on chemotherapy for a year and four months. According to the research, I still had a long way to go.

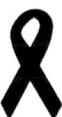

"All Hell Breaks Loose"

In November 2004 Ed and I made one last trip to Florida as snowbirds. We had decided to relocate to New York on a full-time basis. We made the decision for a couple of reasons, one of them being my health. We knew that the cancer could take a turn for the worse at any time. We wanted to make sure that we were close to family and friends if that should happen.

We couldn't afford to pay rent on an apartment in New York while maintaining a boat that was getting older, and in need of work. FREEDOM II had been the perfect boat for us while we were living aboard, but it was a big boat to use just for weekend sails. Also, with my bones hurting, I would not be able to help Ed as much as I used to. All of the maintenance would fall on him. With a great deal of sadness, we made the difficult decision to sell FREEDOM II and get a smaller boat.

In a matter of months we found an apartment in Oakdale on Long Island, sold the boat, and sailed her into New York Harbor for the new owner. We drove to Florida, packed up our belongings, rented a truck, drove back to New York, moved into our new apartment, bought a new car, bought a new boat, drove back to Florida, and trailered the boat home.

We knew that the added expense of living in New York, along with inflation, would put a financial squeeze on our fixed income, so we re-opened Ed's psychotherapy practice, which he had retired from thirteen years earlier. We rented an office, bought office equipment, and got very busy learning how to work with managed care as providers of mental health services. The months from November 2004 through March 2005 were grueling. We were both physically and emotionally exhausted.

Ed's reputation had survived thirteen years of retirement. Many of the agencies that had referred clients to him in the past remembered him and said that they were glad to have him back. By May his practice was running at full capacity. We were starting to settle into our new lifestyle. I was starting to feel strong again. I was starting to find that "old me" that I had been desperate to find.

We spent the last half of the summer enjoying our new sailboat, a 21' trimaran that Ed named PASSING WIND. Life seemed to be back on track. My cancer was still there, but it was responding well to treatment. We had it under control...or so we thought.

August 2005 was most definitely the worst month of my life. I had told my oncologist that I was experiencing pain in my hips and in my spine. He ordered blood to be drawn and tested, and he gave me prescriptions for a PET scan and a bone scan. The results were not good.

The scans showed that the cancer was progressing again. The blood work showed that the cancer marker, which had been within the normal range for over a year, was elevated. It had jumped from 34 to 56.

Between my symptoms, the scans, and the blood levels, we knew that the Femara was no longer working. My oncologist told me that I didn't have to go back on chemo just yet. He wanted to try me on a medication called Faslodex. Faslodex is a hormone treatment for hormone receptor positive metastatic breast cancer. It is for postmenopausal women whose disease had progressed after taking another hormone treatment. I fit all the criteria, so I started the treatment that day. Treatment with Faslodex consisted of an injection in the hind- quarters once a month. The oncologist said that he would monitor my symptoms and my blood work to see how well the treatment was working. I would also remain on Lupron and Zometa.

One month later my blood level had increased again. It was 63. The oncologist told me not to be alarmed. It could be that my body needed time to adjust to the new treatment. He took more blood work. I would have to wait another week before getting the results.

In the meantime, another medical crisis entered our lives. After going for a routine physical in June, Ed learned that his PSA was elevated. The normal range is 1-4. Ed's was 8. (We were learning to live our lives by numbers, blood levels and markers.)

He went to a urologist. He told us that the elevated number could be due to an enlarged prostate. He put Ed on a medication called Flomax and told him to come back in one month.

It was July. My parents celebrated their 50th wedding anniversary by taking the whole family, (all 18 of us), on a 7-day cruise to Bermuda. Unfortunately, Ed had a hard time enjoying himself. He was extremely tired most of the time. He kept saying that he "didn't feel right". Knowing Ed, and his love of the water, I knew that something was wrong. It was terribly unusual for him to be on the ocean and choose to rest in the cabin rather than stay on deck to enjoy the experience. Ed's a sailor. He built his own boat when he was only 10 years old. He has often said that he's happiest when he's <u>on</u> the water, <u>in</u> the water or <u>under</u> the water. He describes the feel of the ocean as, "laying on Mother Nature's belly and feeling her breathe". It scared me to see him so indifferent to this experience.

Some of my family commented on the fact that Ed wasn't acting right. I knew that it was true, and so did Ed. He kept telling me that he had no energy and that he didn't feel good. He just wanted to rest.

After the cruise we returned to the urologist for another PSA test. It came back higher than the first. It was now at 14. The doctor said that Ed would need to have an MRI of his lower spine and hips. He said that he would also need to have a biopsy to test the prostate for cancer.

CANCER!!!

I can't tell you what it felt like to hear that word after all that we had been through. I no longer had my naïve innocence of believing that bad things only happen to other people. I never would have dreamed that one day I would be diagnosed with cancer, but I was. I couldn't imagine Ed being diagnosed as well. It seemed highly unlikely that both of us would have this horrible disease. Still, I was scared. I tried very hard to put my fear aside. I put on my "brave face", took Ed by the hand and told him, "Whatever <u>you</u> have, <u>we</u> have."

Ed received the phone call on a Tuesday afternoon. I was only able to hear his side of the conversation, but I could tell that the news was not good. After hanging up the phone, he told me what the doctor said. Ed was diagnosed with advanced, aggressive prostate cancer that had already spread to his bones. The news hit me like a ton of bricks. I felt as stunned, lost and confused as I had been three years ago when I was first diagnosed. All of the feelings that I had worked so hard to put behind me came bubbling to the surface. Anger. Fear. Frustration. It seemed horribly unfair for both of us to have this disease. I felt cheated in every way imaginable; emotionally, physically, financially, spiritually, and socially. In the past 3 years I had lost my hair, my body image, and my old sense of who I was. I had lost my energy, my ability to exercise, my interest in writing, and my interest in sex. I had lost my ability to be athletic, and my ability to sleep through the night. I had started to take a yoga class, but due to the pain in my bones, I had to give that up. I had started to teach a creative writing class, but due to a lack of energy, I had to give that up too. I had lost my home in Florida. I had lost my boat, and the lifestyle that living on a boat provided me. I had lost so much. I wasn't ready to lose my husband.

After the initial shock subsided, Ed and I talked about the fact that we could also lose an important part of our income. If he became unable to work, we wouldn't be able to afford much of what we had. We would need to give up the new boat, the new apartment, and the new lifestyle that we had just settled into.

I asked Ed if he wanted me to cancel his clients for the evening. He said, "No. Whatever this takes from me it's going to have to take. I'm not giving anything to it." He was handling the news better than I was.

In the following weeks I became very depressed. Along with depression came guilt. I felt guilty for feeling sorry for myself when there were so many people who had it worse than I did. I didn't have children to care for while trying to fight this disease. I didn't have a full time job. I knew that there were many people who did. What right did I have to complain? I felt guilty because I couldn't give Ed's cancer the care and attention that he had given mine. I wanted to support him as he had supported me, but I wasn't sure that I had it in me to do that. I felt guilty for being depressed. I felt depressed for feeling guilty. My emotions were all over the place. I knew it was perfectly normal for me to feel depressed, outraged, guilty, afraid, hurt, disappointed and frustrated, but I hated having those feelings. As a Social Worker

I had spent a great deal of time talking with people about accepting their feelings without judging them as right or wrong. I knew that my feelings were appropriate considering what I was dealing with, but that didn't make it any easier.

It would be a number of weeks before I would be able to give myself permission to feel the anger and the sadness without guilt or shame. I let myself feel cheated. I acknowledged the fact that I had been dealt a difficult hand. I told myself to stop <u>thinking</u> about how to feel, and just go ahead and <u>feel</u>. I let myself feel the hurt. I tried to stop worrying about the future. I acknowledged the fact that bad times, like good times, come and go. We would get through this.

Given that Ed and I both had advanced cancer, I knew that I needed to prepare for the inevitable bad times, appreciate the good times, and accept the fact that cancer would be a constant challenge in our lives.

I decided that since there were certain things I couldn't do anymore because of the pain in my bones, I would pursue other interests and hobbies like painting and drawing. I knew that I would always miss the activities that I had come to love, but focusing on the past and on my limitations was pointless. I needed to let cancer know that it wasn't going to control my actions, my emotions, or my life. As the saying goes, "It's not what happens to you in life, but what you choose to think and do about what happens to you that counts".

Ed's urologist told him that he would begin treatments with Lupron, (the same hormone that I was taking). In my case, the Lupron shut down the estrogen that the cancer cells were feeding on. In Ed's case, the Lupron would shut down his testosterone. He had his first shot on September 9th. We would have to wait 4 months before we would know if the treatment was working.

On December 30, Ed had more blood drawn. The following week we met with the urologist. He gave us good news. The PSA had gone down to 1.7. That meant that the Lupron was working. Ed's cancer was responding to the treatment. To say that we were relieved would be the understatement of the year. Four months had been a long time to hold our breath. Ed received his second shot of Lupron. We left the office, took a deep breath, and got ready to hold it for another four months.

At the same time, we were waiting for the results of my most recent blood work. We prayed that my news would be as good as Ed's.

I called the oncology office and asked for the results of my tests. The nurse called back within the hour and told me that my numbers had gone up again. The good news was that they had only gone up by a small amount. My cancer marker had gone from 34, to 56, then up to 63. It was now at 67. During my last visit, the oncologist told me that the Faslodex might take a while to get into my system. He told me that the small increase in the markers should not alarm me. The fact that the intervals were getting less could be a sign that the medication might be starting to work.

We were 12 days into the New Year. Although we had reason to be optimistic about both of our conditions and their treatments, we never felt that we could totally relax. Cancer was in our lives. We were on the ultimate roller coaster ride of ups and downs, and unpredictable twists and turns. There was no way to tell how long the treatments would work. There was no way to know if, or when, we would find out that the cancer was spreading. There was no way to know how long either of us had to live. Of course, no one knows how long they are going to live. It's just that with cancer, you tend to think about it more often and more seriously. We accepted the fact that the rest of our lives would be filled with tests, waiting, praying, and coping day to day.

I also learned to accept the fact that, at some point, I will have to go back on chemotherapy. This acceptance did not come easy. For a long time I was angry. For a long time I was envious of people who were healthy, and those who were diagnosed with early stage cancers, have chemo, and then go on with their lives. To be perfectly honest, I still have those feelings from time to time. I still get angry. I still get scared. I still get frustrated. However, I have learned to accept these feelings, and in accepting them, they have lost their power over me. This experience with cancer has made me a stronger person. It's helped me to realize that I am capable of facing difficult challenges without falling apart.

Maybe cancer is a blessing in a very...VERY good disguise. I have always believed that there is purpose behind everything that happens to us. Bad things DO happen to good people. There is a lesson in all of life's adversities. Our "job" is to focus on the lessons that the bad things have been brought into our lives to teach us. The lessons are there, we just need to find them.

Being told that I have a life-threatening illness has taught me to slow down and take one day at a time. I am learning that each and every moment is a precious gift. Each and every moment is all that I am guaranteed.

This experience has caused me to take a long, hard, and honest look at my life. What has my life been about? Has my life had purpose and meaning? What have I meant to those around me? What have the significant people in my life meant to me?

Too often we wait until we have lost something, to appreciate the value that it had. I didn't want to live my life that way. I wanted to become more aware of the positive people, places and things in my life, and start showing my gratitude for having them.

I started to think about patterns in my life that had influenced the decisions I'd made, and shaped the woman that I'd become. I started to think about poor judgments that I'd had at certain times in my life, and the mistakes that I had made. I started to think about relationships and opportunities that I did not pursue because of a lack of confidence. I also started to think about all of the good fortune that I had been blessed with throughout my life.

As I reflected upon these significant times, I realized that all of the fun, the mistakes, missed opportunities, and poor decisions had served a purpose. They brought me to this present moment armed with the ability to handle disappointment and adversity. They prepared me to face this battle against cancer by making me a stronger person. They taught me the importance of making the most of the time that I have. They taught me about friendship, love and tolerance. They taught me about being sensitive and caring towards others. They taught me that everything happens for a reason. They taught me that no moment is truly lost as long as you learn a lesson from it.

I am dedicating the rest of my life, however long that may be, to living by the valuable lessons that I have learned through this experience. In this way, no matter what the outcome of this journey is for me, I will have the satisfaction of knowing that I fought it with everything I had and became a better person for it. Although cancer has taken so much from me, it has given me something in return. My experience with cancer has given me a stronger connection to the very life that it threatens to take away.

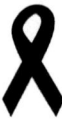

Lessons Learned

Love yourself and others with no conditions and no judgments.

Accept differences in people. We are all different, and that is a wonderful thing.

Stop at various times of the day to consciously capture the energy of the moment.

Have fun and be childlike.

Look for the good in yourself and others.

Relax. Don't take yourself so seriously.

Spend as much time as possible in nature.

Let go of grudges.

Jealousy and envy are useless emotions.

Be kind and gentle with yourself and others.

Don't spread rumors.

Always tell the truth.

Learn to forgive yourself and others.

Learn to express love.

Allow yourself to be loved.

Make the most of your talents and abilities.

Make good decisions.

Remember that sometimes the smallest gestures make the biggest difference.

Always make time in your life for the people you love.

Create your life. Live your life.
Love your life.

Acknowledgements

To my friends and family,

Thank you for all of your inspirational cards, letters, e-mails and phone calls. Thank you for the meals you cooked, the jokes you told, and the prayers you offered in my name. Your love and support has helped me stay strong and determined in my battle against cancer and in the writing of this book. Thank you to my Mother and Father, Loretta and Jimmy Quintana, George and Mary Parisi, Grace and Paul Pedretti, Amy and Ricky Barone, Marcia and Bernie Schwartz, Peter, Rosemarie, Peter, Susan and John Fiorentino, Don and Sharon Stryjewski, Paul Gould and Jen Fox, Dr. Aimée Gould Shunney, Denise and Roger Medved-Belford, Diane and Joe Patenaude, Karen and Sean Von Braunsberg, Sam and Amy Cauley, Susan, Edward, Dylan and Diana Dematteis, Barry and Laurie Rosen, Tom Cavallo and Lili Hughes.

Thank you to Katie, Allison, Jamie, Anthony, Christopher, Teresa, Kara and Valerie for making me the proudest Aunt in the world.

Thank you to all of my friends in W.O.R.C.

Thank you to Rosemary Cavallo for always being with me.

I would specifically like to thank the following people who, at different times and in different ways, helped DEAR CANCER become a reality: Amy Barone, Elisa Holland, Katie Quintana, Loretta Quintana, Sharon Stryjewski, Tom Dyar and the staff at Author House.

My heartfelt gratitude to Dr. Kenneth Gold and Dr. Nicholas Iannotti for not only treating my cancer, but for always treating <u>me</u> with sensitivity, dignity and respect.

Thank you to all of the nurses and staff at Hematology/ Oncology Associates of Western Suffolk and Martin Memorial Cancer Center.

To my husband, Ed, thank you for coming with me to every doctor, lab, and hospital appointment. Thank you for holding me when I needed to cry, encouraging me when I was feeling down, and giving me space when I needed to be alone. Thank you for reading DEAR CANCER over and over (and over) again, and giving me your valuable suggestions. You are my best friend. I want you to know that I never have and never will take your love for granted. We've been through so much together that it's hard to remember a time when we weren't "Edaura". In the words of Jimmy Buffet, "Honey, it's been a lovely cruise." I love you now and always.

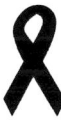

About The Author

Laura Parisi King is a Licensed Master Social Worker. She is the author of GRANDA, a young adult novel about stereotypes and self-discovery. Her short stories have appeared in LISTEN magazine, and she has been a contributor to COPING magazine. Laura has been a creative writing instructor, and she has been a columnist for the newsletter, TAKING THE FEAR OUT OF CANCER. Laura has been interviewed on radio and television and she has been the guest speaker in schools in Florida and New York.

Most importantly, Laura Parisi King is a wife, daughter, sister, niece, aunt, cousin and friend.

Laura spent 5 years living full time aboard a 32-foot catamaran sailboat named FREEDOM II. Along with Ed, her husband and captain, she sailed over 21,000 miles visiting the Florida Keys, the Bahamas and other communities along the East Coast of the United States.

On October 9, 2002 Laura was diagnosed with stage IV breast cancer that had spread to both of her lungs, her ribs, sternum, hips, spine and neck.

Laura knows that, to date, there is no cure for stage IV breast cancer. Her belief is that the mind is a powerful compliment to chemotherapy and other drugs when it comes to battling cancer. That belief led her to write DEAR CANCER. Her hope is that, through her writings, she can bring a sense of strength, a sense of hope, and a sense of support to people with cancer and other life-changing illnesses and events.

Laura and Ed currently live in Oakdale, New York.

Printed in the United States
55478LVS00005B/274-351